OLD AGE

D1880958

Owing to the antiquity and rarity of this book, certain pages are regrettably absent, and readability is compromised due to the blurring of the original text. If you possess any insights regarding the availability of these missing sections, kindly inform us. Your assistance is crucial in ensuring the completion of this significant work for the benefit of future generations.

OLD AGE

ITS CAUSE AND PREVENTION

FILIPPO DE FILIPPI

GYAN

Published by

GYAN

Gyan Publishing House
5, Ansari Road
Daryaganj, New Delhi-110002
Phone: 011-47034999, 9811692060
E-mail: books@gyanbooks.com

Distribution Network
gyanbooks.com
India, USA, Canada, UK, Australia

© Publisher

All rights reserved. No part of this work may be reproduced, stored, adapted, or transmitted in any form or by any means, electronic, mechanical, photocopying, micro-filming, recording or otherwise, or translated in any language, without the prior written permission of the copyright owner and the publisher.

ISBN: 978-93-7225-309-2 (PB)

First Published, 1912

2nd Impression 2026

Printed at: Gyan Press, Delhi.

The book is sold subject to the condition that it shall not, by way of trade or otherwise, be lent, resold, hired out, or otherwise circulated without the prior publisher's written consent.

OLD AGE

Author: FILIPPO DE FILIPPI

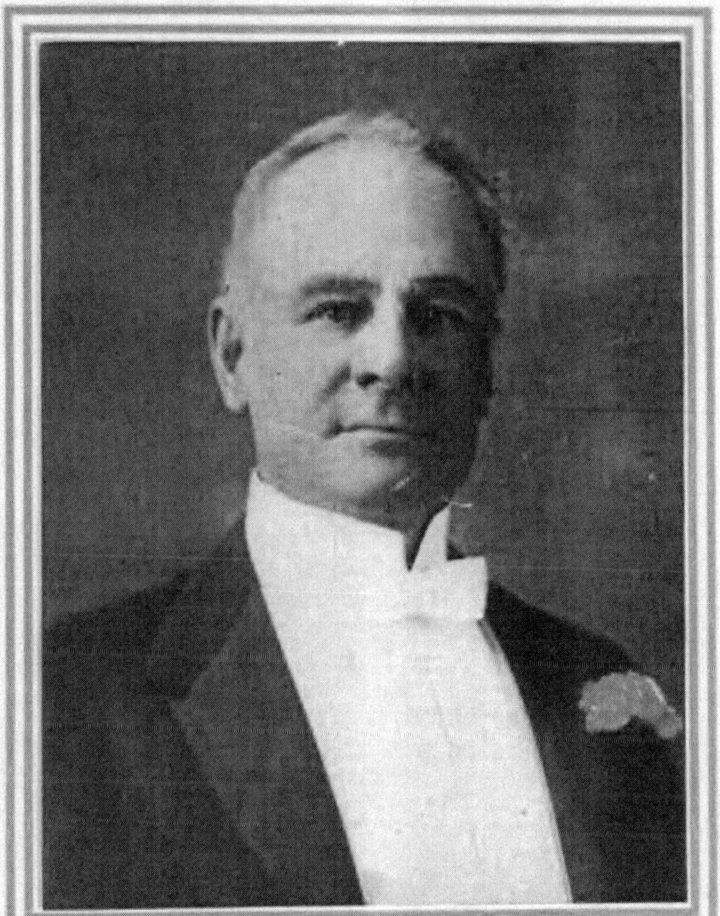

SANFORD BENNETT AT SEVENTY-TWO YEARS OF AGE
SAN FRANCISCO, CAL., JANUARY 4th, 1912

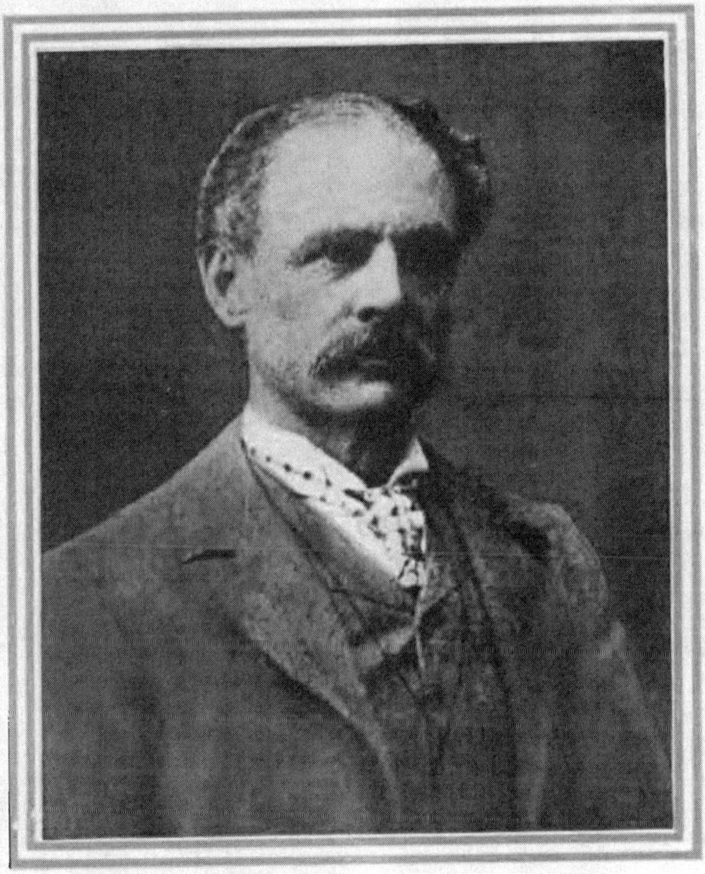

SANFORD BENNETT AT FIFTY YEARS OF AGE
SAN FRANCISCO, CAL., JUNE 8th, 1889

ALL MUSCLES AND ALL ORGANS INCREASE IN SIZE, STRENGTH AND ELASTICITY WHEN PROPERLY EXERCISED. THIS IS THE PRINCIPAL SECRET OF HEALTH, STRENGTH, ELASTICITY OF BODY, AND A LONG LIFE

OLD AGE

ITS CAUSE AND PREVENTION

THE STORY OF AN OLD BODY
AND FACE MADE YOUNG

BY SANFORD BENNETT

"THE MAN WHO GREW YOUNG AT SEVENTY"
AUTHOR OF "EXERCISING IN BED"

PUBLISHED BY
THE PHYSICAL CULTURE PUBLISHING CO.
NEW YORK CITY, U. S. A.

Copyrighted, 1912, by
SANFORD BENNETT

I DEDICATE THIS BOOK TO MY

DAUGHTER,

MY FIRST PUPIL IN THE GREATEST OF ALL

SCIENCES: THE SCIENCE OF

HEALTH

Contents

PAGE

Illustrations

PAGE

From 1841 to 1912

ALL statements presented in this book are based upon my successful personal experiences in the art of physical rejuvenation in advanced years, and this success is the result of long and persistent investigation of the causes of physical old age and the practice of Nature's methods for its prevention. These investigations, combined with twenty-five years of experiments upon my own body, have taught me how to postpone that unpleasant condition.

I am not theorizing or writing the experiences of some one else, but verify the truth of my statements by my own youthful physical condition at seventy-two. If my case was simply one of physical preservation in advanced years, other instances would be cited equally unusual, but mine is not a case of physical preservation. It is one of physical acquisition or of acquiring the elasticity, strength and health characteristic of youth "at three score and ten," an age when such improvement has hitherto been supposed to be impossible.

At fifty I was physically an old man. Many years of a too active business career had resulted in a general break-down. I was then wrinkled, partially bald, cheeks sunken, face drawn and haggard, muscles atrophied, and thirty years of chronic dyspepsia finally resulted in catarrh of the stomach, with acid rheumatism periodically adding its agonies. I was an old man and looked it. It was the desperation of my case which induced me to undertake these experiments. I have made many mistakes which it has required time to rectify, but the desire to live has impelled me to struggle on and finally I have succeeded. But the road to that success has not been easy, as lacking experienced guides, I had to pioneer my own way over a road that proved to be long and difficult. Another great obstacle was, that the customs of my short-lived family could not be readily abandoned. If any of us were sick we promptly "took something for it," something which we bought at a drug store. In my many sicknesses as a child I have had an intimate acquaintance with apparently most alleged medicinal remedies—anything my anxious relatives could think of, or an allopathic family physician advised.

It is a depressing list to look back upon. It ranges from "Adams Calomel Pills" to "Zeehandlers World Renowned Fever and Ague Cure." But I think I have sampled them all. Naturally, I grew up with a firm belief that in medicines lay the only curative process, and I regarded drug stores as life-saving stations.

I remained in that belief until I had reached the age of fifty, and—broke down. The enumeration of my physical woes at that age is a truthful statement of the conditions then existing. And now in my seventy-second year I present the healthy conditions of an athlete in training and the appearance of a man of little more than half of my years. Under these conditions my success is too obvious to be overlooked. The fact is—unacceptable as it may be to the vast numbers of the medical profession, and also to the industries connected with it—I succeeded only after I had discontinued all medicines. Health cannot be found in drug store prescriptions, nor can life be materially prolonged by any medical preparations. The solution of the problem lies only in Nature's principal methods of inducing health—sunlight, pure air, pure water, nourishing food, cleanliness and exercise. Given these most important factors and an observance of what we know as the general laws of hygiene, health and a long life are possible, and usually very probable. But without these conditions, they are not obtainable and the long category of medicinal remedies with which the world has been afflicted will not replace such conditions.

What I have accomplished is possible to almost any one who is not organically so wrong as to be hopeless. But to the average man or woman whose condition is simply that of general physical deterioration, termed "old age," I extend this message of hope: Follow my example and success will be yours. I have been an old man, and now at over "three score and ten" I am a young man again, and look it. Really, I am now a younger man physically than I was in the best period of my early manhood, say at thirty-five. In some respects, I seem to have accomplished the fabled miracle of Faust as to a considerable extent I have transformed an old body into a young one, and this without the aid of Faust's friend, or any supplies obtained from his extremely popular medical departments.

As I have said, I have been compelled to find the right path alone, for although I read extensively upon the matter of which I write, I never found a satisfactory guide book to the goal I sought; that is, one based upon the author's authenticated personal experiences. A part of the way is clearly shown by Lewis Cornaro, a Venetian nobleman who lived to the age of one hundred years, dying at Padua April 26th, 1566. The title of that book is, "Sure and Certain Methods of Attaining A Long and Healthy Life." But you will find the same dietetic rules more clearly explained in almost any health book, especially in Horace Fletcher's works. The point of interest is that the author, Lewis Cornaro, proved the truth of his statements by his own personal experiences. And that is just what I have done, as I shall tell you how in this book. My statements of the methods by which I succeeded will therefore be of interest.

I have found many well-authenticated cases of persons who have lived nearly to the limit of human life, that is, one hundred years; several who have reached that period, but no authenticated instance of any human being who, in advanced years (say after the age of fifty or sixty), had regained to any considerable degree the physical conditions and appearance of youth. Counterfeits, yes, but like all counterfeits, detection finally resulted. "A man is as old as his arteries" is a well-worn truism, to which may be added, that woman is sometimes seemingly as young as her artifices would make her appear. But that condition is unsatisfactory and easily detected by other women, who, as a rule, are usually experts in that direction. But when you become young by the methods I practice, you will pass muster under the most searching investigation. At least, that has been my experience with the various clinical examinations of my body by the most able surgeon I could find. More superficial examinations by other interested scientists have also been frequently made, but always with the same result. My trouble now is, that while all who see me agree that I look but little more than half my age, they express doubt that I am in my seventy-second year.

There is little difficulty in proving that I was born in Philadelphia, Pa., January 4th, 1841. Therefore, I reached my seventy-second birthday upon the fourth day of January, 1912. Furthermore, I have a kind of dubious war record, which is not difficult to verify, not a very brilliant one, I must admit, but I don't regret it. In 1861 I occupied for a time the position of bookkeeper and general clerk for the regimental sutler or storekeeper attached to the "Baxter Zouaves" regiment of Philadelphia. We were stationed at Harper's Ferry, Virginia. That regiment participated in the disastrous battle of Ball's Bluff, fought across the river at that point. The date of that bloody action was October 21st, 1861. I probably saved my life by staying with the stores upon the safe side of the river. Therefore, I took no part in the fight and am glad I did not. We were all "three months' men," and when at the end of our term of service a lot of us were permitted to go home, I promptly availed myself of the chance, and went. Incidentally, I would remark that I would have gone sooner if I could. That is why, very probably, I have missed the glory upon Decoration Day, of being one of the nation's honored dead. To the best of my recollection I was a battle-scarred veteran only to the extent of my baggy red pants and silver-buttoned jacket. That is my war record. It has nothing to do with my system of physical rejuvenation, but verifies my age. I was then a young man of twenty-one and I occupied a responsible position which could not have been filled by a boy.

The truth of my statement regarding my age being admitted, the next explanation of my physical rejuvenation, always advanced by outsiders, is that I must be abnormally endowed with the vital principle. This is also a mistake. My father died of consumption at the age of forty-two, a nervous, dyspeptic man, always ailing, and always "taking something for it." But through it all, he was an energetic, successful business man; his goal, financial success; health, a secondary consideration; the result, death at forty-two. The same type of man you see everywhere in all large cities. I inherited my father's physical disabilities and also, to a great extent, his characteristics. With such hereditary tendencies I came into this life January 4th, 1841, a sickly little nervous shred of a child, whom no one ever expected to live through childhood, and to whom reaching maturity seemed an impossibility. But "there is a Divinity that shapes our ends, rough hew them as we will," and now at seventy-two, I realize that my mission in this life must be to show others Nature's simple methods of health, and how by their observance our stay here may be prolonged and lost physical youth may be regained, this, at an age when such improvement has heretofore been supposed to be impossible.

These were the unfavorable conditions of my feeble childhood, and throughout my boyhood the haunting spectre of consumption was ever present.

Following my father's example I engaged in mercantile pursuits, and the conduct of my business life was similar to his, similar to that of all high-pressure business men in this country. Then at fifty, worried and worn out with the financial cares of a great mercantile industry, suffering from lack of exercise, hurried meals and a "no-time-to-spare" life, I collapsed. The brink of the precipice had been reached. A month's enforced rest gave me ample time to think over the discouraging situation. Then I woke up to the realization that I was almost a subject for Osler's chloroform treatment. I decided to turn over a new leaf. What I did is set forth in this book.

This summary of my life will dispose of the suggestion of favorable environment or favorable physical antecedents. We are not a long-lived family, either upon my father's or mother's side. They have all long ago solved the great mystery—father, mother, sister, brother, uncles and aunts all gone.

Under these conditions my start in life

cannot be said to have been favorable. There is still another question to be answered. That is: Might not my unprecedented return to the conditions of youth be a case of atavism, that some one of my long forgotten ancestors had been an instance of the same phenomena I present? When at sixty I found that I was certainly growing younger, that question also presented itself to me. I therefore thoroughly investigated the antecedents of my family and its branches for nearly two hundred years. The result of that search evidenced the fact that I am not descended from a long-lived race, nor are there any instances of its individuals who have lived to an unusual age.

As a summary of the matter it is therefore evident, that my unprecedented physical rejuvenation at seventy-two is not due to any hereditary advantage, favorable environments or physical peculiarity.

Narrowing the investigation, it becomes evident that such rejuvenation was either due to some method of life, article of food, or medicinal preparation. As to the latter, my views have been so frequently and decidedly expressed as to at once eliminate that hypothesis. Regarding any rational system of diet being a means of health, decidedly yes, but that any dietary system alone or any article of food could have produced the results which I have accomplished is impossible.

The term of our stay upon this earth is surely influenced by the food taken to sustain life. But I am an omnivorous individual. I eat whatever I like and perhaps eat too much, as I have a small-boy appetite. Furthermore, I have some bad habits and as I am upon the witness stand I will confess that I smoke a little and usually drink beer or claret at my meals, but only then. I never take either whiskey or brandy, as the percentage of alcohol contained in either is too great and both have a speedy and very bad effect upon me. And when I find anything disagrees with me, or any particular way of life is hurtful, I don't go that way, or at least, with caution, and to a very limited extent. The light claret and small amount of beer I drink seems to agree with me and while the one mild post-prandial cigar I smoke per diem is, I think, a bad and inadvisable habit, I do not, as yet, find any evil effect from it. If I did, then that habit would at once be discontinued.

After this confession of my various shortcomings, small opinion of alleged infallible medicinal remedies and an evident inattention to a strict dietary regime, the question will naturally arise: Then what is the method by which I have transformed an old, worn-out body into an elastic, healthy and to all appearances, a young one? That is the subject of subsequent chapters.

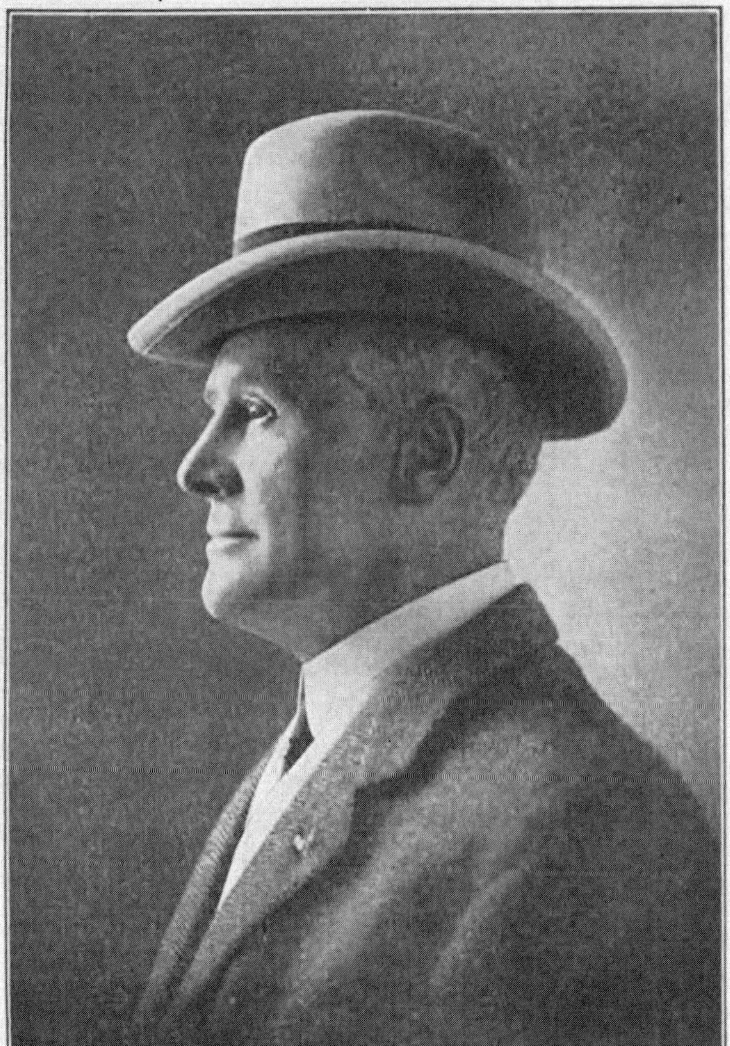

SANFORD BENNETT AT 72
Note the smooth throat lines

Why I Have Written This Book

THIS book is a record of my own personal experience in the art of Physical Rejuvenation, with a clear account of the methods by which, at the age of seventy-two, I have thrown off the conditions of age, and have become, physically, a young man again. And this has been accomplished without the use of medicinal preparations of any nature. What has been possible in my case is, most probably, just as possible in yours. The methods by which I have made this success have the advantage of being without cost, and as the directions for the exercises I practice are so clearly described and illustrated, you will need no other instructor than this book. There are no technical or scientific names to puzzle you, therefore you will readily comprehend that which follows:

The muscular contractions and alternate relaxations of every muscle of the body, which are the basis of this system, are all performed while lying in bed. Hence, the title "Exercising in Bed," given to my former publications upon the subject. The methods I describe will, if persistently and methodically practiced, result in improved circulation, healthy glandular activity, and materially prolong your life. My own case of physical rejuvenation at over "three score and ten" has attracted a great deal of attention, and has been very extensively commented upon by the press, the articles generally appearing under the caption of "The Man Who Grew Young At Seventy."

Attracted by these numerous "write ups" and the simplicity of my methods of physical culture, others have followed my example and now that "Exercising in Bed" has reached the sixth edition, a great many people are practicing these exercises and are enthusiastic converts to this "lazy man's" system of obtaining health, and getting young again. As a consequence, I have been the recipient of a great mass of letters, and many valuable suggestions.

My ability for stealing, and then adapting, to my own purposes, the good ideas of other people, combined with my own personal experiences, has resulted in the really valuable book I now present, the title of which is, OLD AGE—ITS CAUSE AND PREVENTION. I believe it to be the best compilation upon the art of Physical Rejuvenation, through Nature's methods, which has yet appeared. Indeed it must be, as after nearly a quarter of a century of constant practicing, reading and experimenting in this direction, I have adapted (stolen, if you will) the best, logical and proven valuable, suggestions of the most able writers upon this subject, and by adding to these valuable suggestions my own successful experience in getting young again, I feel confident that after reading it you will agree with me when I declare that "this is a valuable book." It is impossible for me to give due credit to all of the authorities whose ideas I have appropriated, after I had demonstrated their value by my own personal experience, and if any of these writers should in this book run across something that is familiar, something for which they feel they should have credit, I will quote the case of the Chicago Pork Packer, who bought a gallery of Ancestral Portraits. "I don't know whose Ancestors they were," said he, "but by Gosh, they're mine now, and I'm going to let 'em have some needed improvements."

Regarding my criticisms upon the antiquated and dangerous allopathic methods of treating disease, the "dose 'em as long as they will stand it" type, I have nothing to retract. From babyhood to the age of fifty, I suffered from those methods and never was a well man until I ceased the habit of "taking something for it" when I was the least indisposed. Now, I am mad all over when I think of that prolonged, distressing experience. Nature does not cure that way and a long, healthy life is not possible by the practice of such antiquated methods. Those who have had the same experience will agree with me. You will find my views upon this matter again and again expressed throughout this book, which is a plea for Nature's methods of cure, therefore a protest against the alleged medicinal "remedies," which so nearly ended my existence. I repeat, that a long and healthy life is not possible by such methods and I never was a healthy man until I realized that fact.

Many of my readers may not wholly agree with me as to the danger of the medicine habit, but anyhow you will find my views upon that matter fully ventilated later on. The "dose 'em" practitioners of the allopathic school of the medical profession, also the drug interests, will undoubtedly say, "the man is a fool, don't know what he is talking about, and both he and his health system are nonsense." To those objectors I will answer as Mrs. Mulligan did to the widow Casey, "You are all that you say I am, and a good deal more that I'm a thinkin'."

The drug prescription and patent medicine business is at present a powerful industry, and if I were personally giving advice either written or verbally for a fee, I would hesitate before "treading upon the coat tails" of such a powerful organization. But I do not "practice," neither have I pupils, classes nor anything to sell, and I propose to keep up my written protest against the stupid, antiquated and harmful methods of drug dosing, allopathic practices, as long as I live. It is all wrong, there is a better way to cure ill-health, and that is the way I show you in this book.

My success in regaining at seventy-two, the health and elasticity of body, characteristic of the condition of healthful youth has been so remarkable that it is absolutely convincing. The annals of medicine cannot show any case in which, by the use of medicines alone, such results have been obtained, and I will add, they never will, and now, at an age past the erroneous Biblical limitation of human life, I realize that my mission here must be to show others the path which has led to my success. That is one of the reasons why I have written this book. There is another and less noble incentive, the same natural desire which prompts the donation of libraries, endowment of hospitals, the installation of stained glass windows in churches, or the insertion of slabs in public buildings, all bearing the donors' names and in many cases, as many of his or her alleged or real virtues as the space will permit. The same instinct which prompts Mr. J. Fitzclarence Kilgubbin, of Oshkosh, U. S. A., to scratch his illustrious name upon the apex of the pyramids or the coat-tails of the Sphinx. Still, I will plead some extenuating circumstances.

In a way, I was compelled to write and publish my experiences in rejuvenation. I came to San Francisco forty years ago, and in the

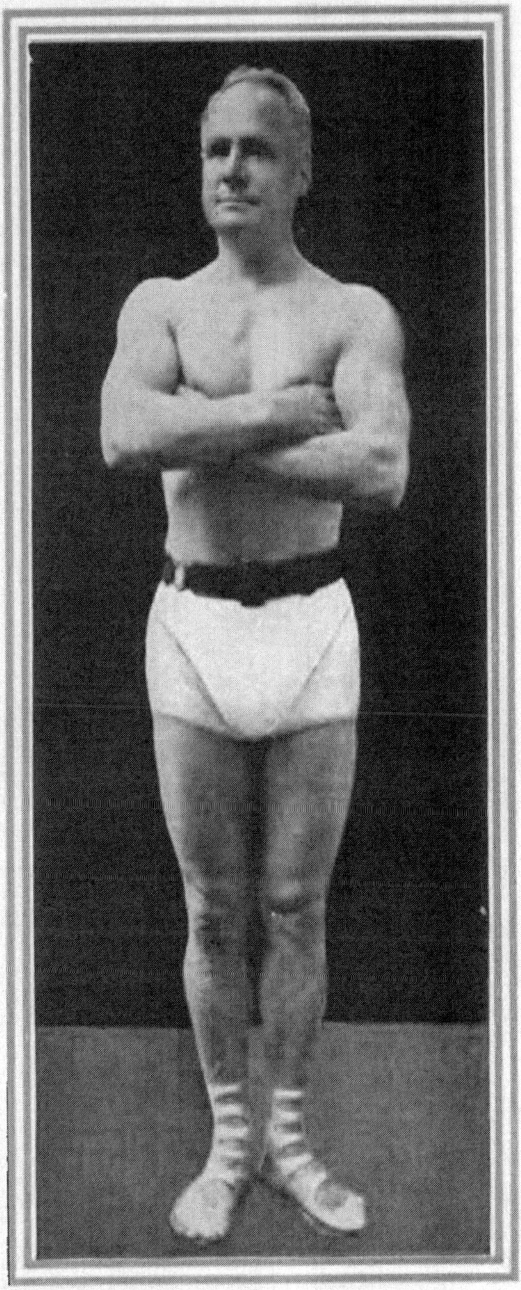

FRONT VIEW SHOWING GENERAL DEVELOPMENT AT SEVENTY-TWO

hurry and worry of business life I became old. Then after the age of fifty I reversed the ordinary course of life and grew young again. This infraction of what, from experience, we know as the usual rule of life, attracted a good deal of attention. Finally I agreed to write for the *San Francisco Chronicle,* a series of articles upon the subject; describing the methods by which I had accomplished my unprecedented rejuvenation. Here is what started the trouble and made me an author:

San Francisco Chronicle, Sunday, November 25th, 1906.

"To the financial, manufacturing and mercantile interests of this city, no man is more widely known than Sanford Bennett. For many years he was Treasurer of the San Francisco Board of Trade, and for over twenty years was Secretary and Treasurer of Dunham Camgan and Hayden Company. At fifty years of age, Mr. Bennett was an old man and looked the part. Today, at the age of sixty-six, he looks to be thirty-five or forty, and feels it."

As for ten months thereafter, I regularly furnished the Sunday *Chronicle* with a series of excellently illustrated articles describing the methods by which I had accomplished my rejuvenation and was extensively "written up" all over the United States and England, the amount of free advertising and correspondence resulting can be readily imagined. I was unable to answer the letters which poured in upon me from all parts of the country. To solve the difficulty I finally assembled the published newspaper matter into book form, adopting the quaint title, "Exercising in Bed," issuing an edition of two thousand copies, as in that way I hoped to answer all questions. That edition was speedily exhausted, but after discovering some mistakes and omissions in that first book, I re-wrote it, using nearly the same title, but with the addition of much new matter.

This last book, published by The Physical Culture Publishing Company, of New York, had a very large sale. It is not possible to improve upon the system of exercises described in "Exercising in Bed," as the muscular contractions and relaxations there described, bring into activity every muscle of the body, therefore, you will find that system of exercise included and fully described and illustrated, in this last literary effort of mine.

Since I commenced writing upon this interesting matter, six years ago, I have, through unremitting study, investigations, and personal experiments, added much valuable information to the matter. Therefore, I believe in OLD AGE—ITS CAUSE AND PREVENTION, you will find data and advice which if considered carefully and followed as I direct, will be of great value to you. The greatest of all sciences is the science of health, which includes the most effective means of prolonging life by Nature's methods.

A large number of letters have been received from ladies, and frequently from the sterner sex, asking my advice as to methods of rejuvenating the face and throat. The information desired will be found in the chapters upon that subject, the exercises I have devised and practiced, therefore, being illustrated and clearly described. You will find them very effective and all of the exercises to the number of thirty, you will find illustrated in the chapter "Exercising in Bed." These exercises have been placed in the order I have found most convenient for practice.

Mechanical devices I no longer use, as I have discovered they are not absolutely necessary for physical development, but as many people insist upon them, and as they appeared in my first publications upon the subject, they are included in this book. The directions and illustrations for these muscular contractions and relaxations are simple and easily understood; therefore, you should not need an instructor, if you will carefully read and remember my directions. As to the proof of my success in the art of rejuvenation in advanced years, I refer you to the portrait which appears on page iii of this book. This photograph was taken upon my seventy-second birthday, January 4th, 1912. Compare it with the picture

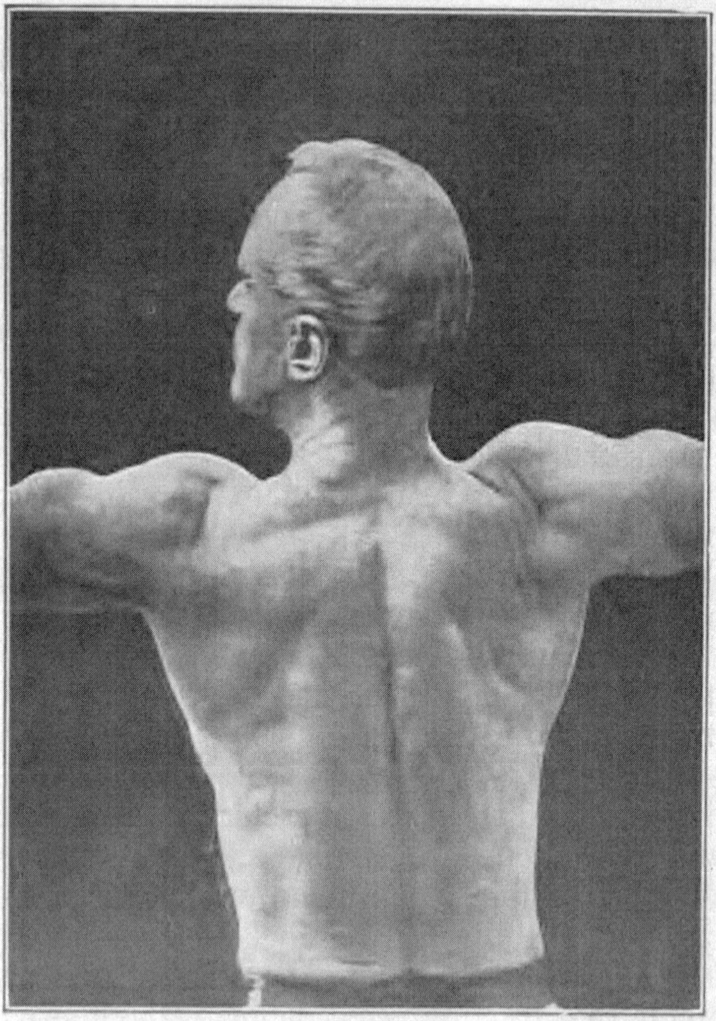

Development of the Shoulders and Muscles of the Back

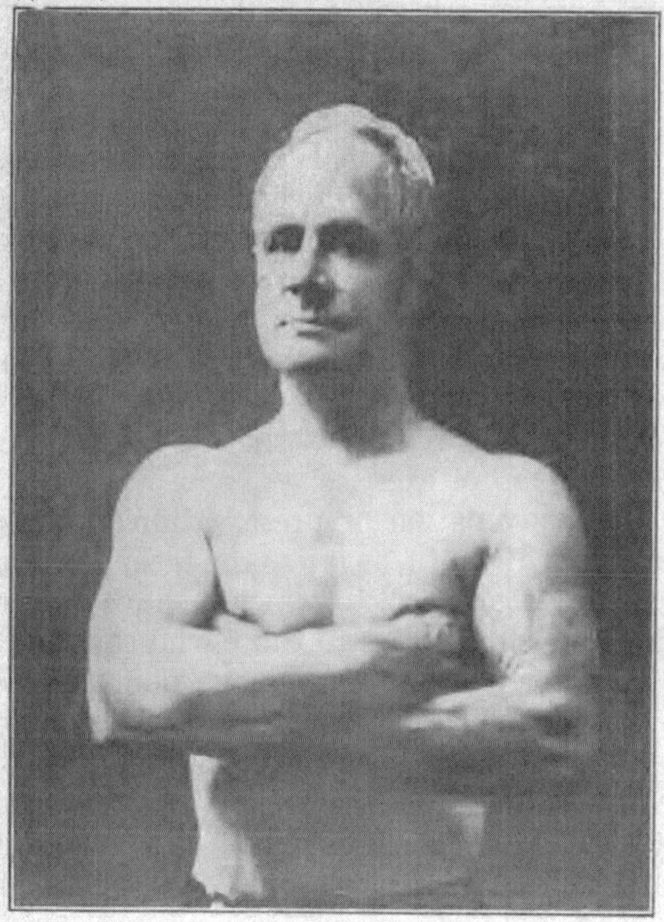

Development of Shoulders and Biceps at Age 72

facing it, which was taken at the age of fifty years. You will then appreciate the possibilities of the system of physical culture rejuvenation described in these pages.

I repeat that I have nothing to sell and must decline giving personal instruction, but feel absolutely certain that what I have done you can do. I practice what I preach and have made a great success of it and so will you if you will carry out my directions. The chapter upon the power of the will in exercise is of the most vital importance; read it carefully. You will find there the key note of success in this or any other system of exercise.

The rejuvenation or preservation of the appearances of youth, as far as the face, throat and neck are concerned, to which I have referred, may seem superfluous to those who consider the matter solely from a hygienic point of view. But the instructions will probably be of interest to all women, for in the exercises and methods described lies the secret of the remarkable physical preservation of Ninon de L'Enclos, the wonderful French beauty, "The Woman Who Never Grew Old."

To a wage earner, either man or woman, they may also commend themselves, as it is an unfortunate fact that the appearance of facial age is a detriment and lessens your value as an employee. Therefore, look young. It may require some time and exertion to do so, but it will pay you. To all men and women I present a system which if followed carefully will surely improve your health and prolong your life. It also has this merit: Nature's methods of cure require no financial expenditure but they are wonderfully effective, as I have demonstrated. The hope that others will follow my example and have the same success is "Why I Have Written This Book."

Clinical Report

By Dr. Carl Renz
966 Sutter Street, San Francisco

Mr. Sanford Bennett, the author of this book, has been the subject of frequent professional examinations during the past eleven years, or, as shown by my office records, first examination made by me February 5th, 1895.

When commencing these periodical examinations, he requested that I should keep a careful record of any changes in his physical condition which I might detect, explaining that he had devised a system of muscular contractions and alternate relaxations, which he practiced as he lay in bed, and which he believed would eliminate the worn-out or dead and clogging cellular tissue, hoping that in this way he could rejuvenate his body, which at that period exhibited the conditions usual after the fiftieth year has been passed. His general appearance was that of a man whose vocation had necessitated an indoor life. The outlines of his first record are:

Height, 5 feet 6 inches.
Weight, 136 pounds.
Abdomen, with decided embonpoint.

Skin, sallow.

Varicose Vein on inside of right leg (uses an elastic stocking).

Neck, 14 inches.

Skin, around throat, hanging loose.

Legs, well developed.

Arm Muscles, atrophied and flabby from lack of exercise.

Forehead, deeply lined.

Hair, thin, dark, streaked with gray on crown; quite bald.

Chest Expansion, 3 inches; symptoms of arteriosclerosis slightly developed.

Hearing and eyesight, good.

Size of Liver, normal.

Heart, normal dimensions; no valvular lesion.

Pulse, about 76; not quite regular.

Lungs, normal.

Complains of Chronic Dyspepsia; is distressed after meals; biliousness; heart palpitations.

Temperament, very nervous.

Urine, without sugar or albumen; of high specific gravity; at times containing uric acid, at others, phosphates.

General physical conditions, poor.

Appearance, that of a man who had devoted much attention to his business, to the neglect of his health.

DR. C. RENZ.

Clinical Examination April 1, 1906

Or After a Lapse of Eleven Years from First Examination.

At this date I find a great change in the condition of the muscles, organs, skin, hair, and general health of the subject, who really seems to be rejuvenated.

The hair, now gray, has become quite luxuriant. No indications of former baldness.

The neck, increased to 15 inches, smooth and very muscular; in appearance, the neck of a young man.

Throat, full.

Skin at this point no longer loose and hanging, but firm.

Chin and cheeks, round.

Face, smooth; color, excellent. Appearance of the face is that of a healthy, well preserved man of forty or less. The lines which formerly existed have disappeared.

The development of the arms, chest, back, shoulders, and abdominal muscles creditable for an athlete of thirty.

Heart, sound; no palpitation or irregularity of pulse.

Chest expansion, $5\frac{1}{4}$ inches.

Waist, 28 inches. No fat around the abdomen; digestion good.

There is a remarkable preservation of tissue integrity and functional activity; the subject has now entered his 66th year, and has all of the elasticity and appearance of a young man.

Under these favorable physical conditions it would be pure speculation to hazard an opinion as to the probable future span of life. The record of my examinations shows a steady improvement of the subject at an age when such improvement is very unusual; this condition seeming to be due solely to the systematic method of muscular contractions and alternate relaxations which he daily practices.

The success which Mr. Bennett has obtained would seem to be a practical verification of the truth of his theory, "that the secret of health, longevity, and elasticity of the body lies solely in the elimination of dead and worn out cellular tissue, which if allowed to remain in the system would impede the functions and shorten life; and that the only method by which this dead cellular matter can be eliminated is by muscular activity."

Dr. C. Renz.

Third Clinical Report of

Dr. Carl Renz, City of Paris Building, San Francisco, Cal., February 15th, 1912.

At this date I do not find any change in the physical condition of Mr. Sanford Bennett, materially differing from my last report of the case made April 1st, 1906. Aside from a very slight degree of arteriosclerosis I do not find any of the senile changes, naturally to be expected at the age of 72, that being the present age of the subject. The face is remarkably smooth and free from wrinkles. The sagging of the cheeks, chin and throat, evident 17 years ago, are no longer present. He has the appearance of an unusually well preserved man of middle age, and his movements evidence an elastic body. The entire muscular structure is remarkably well developed. He has a normal digestion. No attention seems to be paid to any particular system of diet, and I regret to say that he pays little regard to my advice not to smoke or overeat. DR. C. RENZ.

I admit the truth of the statement of Dr. Renz as to my bad habits, but as I confidently expect to be 100 years old, and as it is well known that "the good die young," I am afraid to shorten my life by being too good. That is the only excuse I can offer for those bad habits, except that I have a ravenous small-boy appetite and thoroughly appreciate a good after-dinner cigar. But Dr. Renz is right, and I am now burning up my last box of cigars, ONE AT A TIME. SANFORD BENNETT.

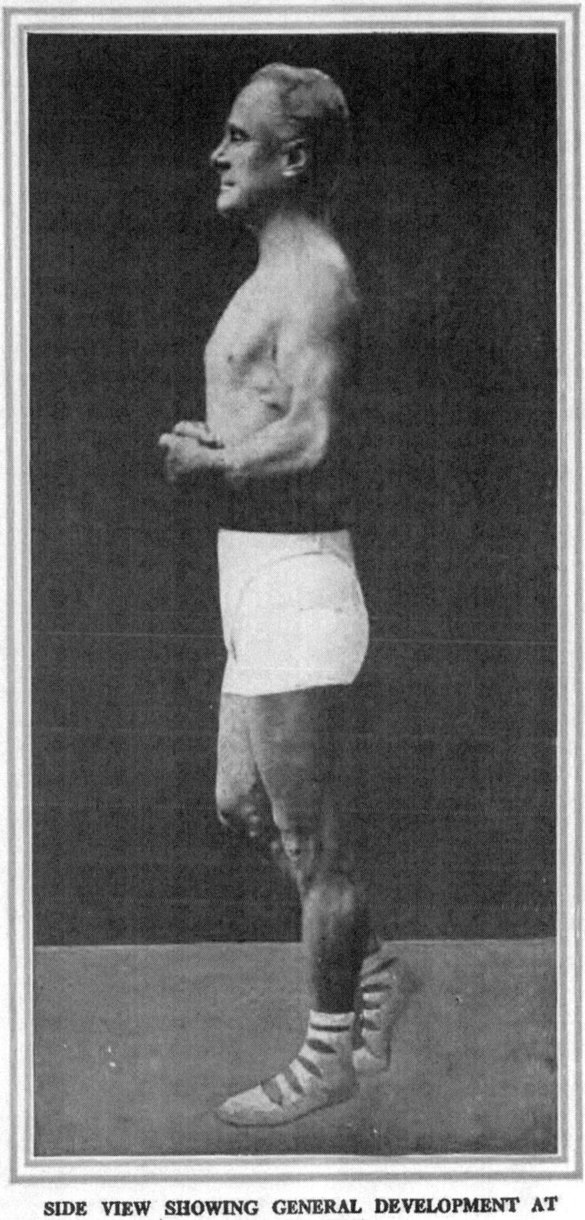

SIDE VIEW SHOWING GENERAL DEVELOPMENT AT SEVENTY-TWO

Old Age—Its Cause and Prevention

WHAT we know as old age is a disease, and like many other diseases it is progressive. For as we advance in years the primal cause increases; this being due to sedimentary deposits in the arterial and venous structures. If the formation of these deposits is not checked, other parts of the system will later directly suffer, and a general physical deterioration indirectly result. Under these conditions, the elasticity of youth gives place to the inelasticity of old age.

The only difference between a young body and an old one seems to be the elasticity of the former and the inelasticity of the latter. Various other causes of age will be cited by scientists who may criticize this statement, but it is undeniable that as we advance in years, these ever increasing deposits result in arteriosclerosis; that is, a clogging up of the arteries by chalky deposits, the final result being general physical deterioration. Under these conditions, the familiar indications of age inevitably appear and we speak of the person so afflicted as an old man or woman. If it is possible to eliminate those sedimentary clogging deposits, the body will regain its elasticity and to a great extent become young again. I am positive from my own personal experience that if in middle life or when indications of chalky deposits first appear, the methods by which I have regained my physical youth, at over three score and ten, are practiced, those symptoms will disappear and physical deterioration caused by them will be greatly retarded.

We cannot finally defy old age, neither can a very old body be transformed into a very young body; but age can certainly be deferred, and the simple means by which I have succeeded in accomplishing this are clearly described in this book. These sedimentary deposits in the system are to some extent similar to the calcareous incrustations which after prolonged use appear in the tubes of a boiler, especially if the water used is heavily charged with lime. If this is the case, they soon become clogged up and unless cleaned are useless, but when cleaned of the clogging matter they again resume their former efficiency. This familiar example will serve to illustrate the condition which takes place in the tubes or arteries of the human body. It is then termed arteriosclerosis. It is a disease of age which can not be cured by any medicinal preparation, neither can those deposits be removed from the body by any system of diet. Theoretically and as a laboratory experiment, it would seem that they can be pre-

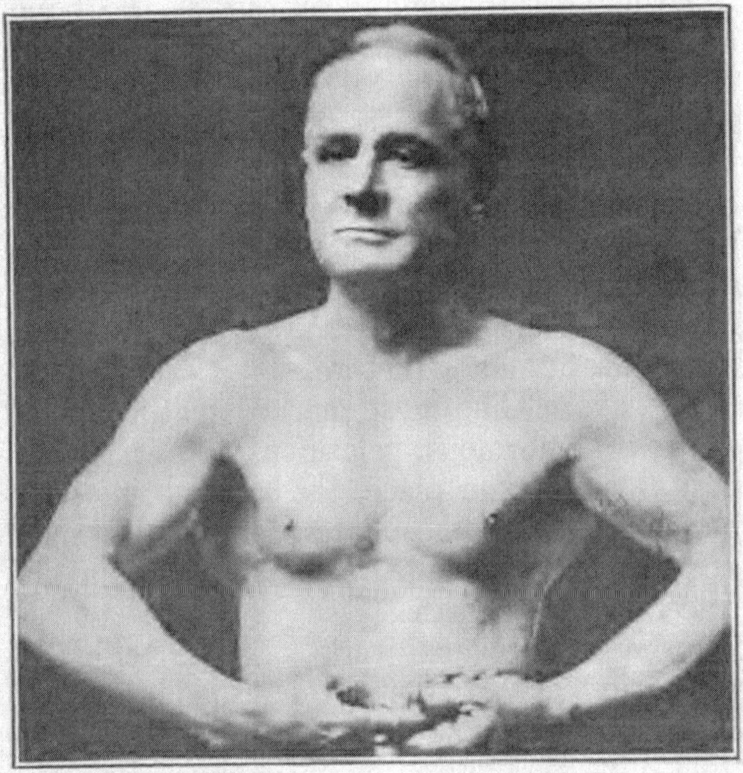

Showing Chest Development at 72

vented by living only upon foods that are slightly charged with lime, but in actual life this is so difficult as to be practically impossible.

To make this clogging process clearer I will quote at length from Dr. De Lacy Evans' interesting work, "How to Prolong Life." While I do not wholly agree with the eminent scientist's views upon certain dietetic methods that he suggests as a means of preventing arteriosclerosis, his description of earthy deposits in the human body is a clear, scientific explanation of their character, also of their effects upon the human structure.

He says: "The most marked feature of old age is that fibrinous, gelatinous and earthy deposits have taken place, the latter being composed chiefly of phosphate of lime with small quantities of sulphate of lime, magnesia and traces of other earths."

From a standard work upon arterial degeneration, by M. Gubler, I also quote: "By anatomic examination it is found that the thickening and induration of the muscular membrane is due to the accumulation of a whitey, yellow, granulous and fatty substance, but essentially of mineral composition, the greater part of which is represented by the carbonate and earthy phosphates. These deposits naturally result in the process of life, and with years, will increase just as the calcareous incrustations form in the boiler tubes, and are just as detrimental to the human mechanism. As a consequence of these deposits the arteries become, in old age, thickened and lessened in caliber. Thus the supply of blood to the brain becomes less and less, its functions are impaired, and the vigorous brain of middle life gradually gives place to the loss of memory, confusion of ideas, inability to follow a long current of thought, carelessness of momentary impression and general imbecility characteristic of old age."

This is a concise summary of the cause of mental deterioration usual in very advanced years. It also applies to the entire muscular and organic structure. Think of the arteries and capillaries as an intricate network of tubes. Through these tubes the blood containing the material required for building your body is conveyed to all parts of the body. In that process there must naturally be sedimentary deposits, and when the tubes become clogged or lessened in caliber, the blood supply to the various organs is insufficient. As a consequence, they deteriorate just as a plant would wither if not properly watered and nourished. And that is old age. As technically described, it is arteriosclerosis, "a filling up and hardening of the arteries." If by any means it is possible to eliminate from the system those clogging deposits and also to prevent their further formation, then the body will again become elastic and the conditions of physical youth return. That this is possible I have demonstrated in my own person, and it is just as possible to you if you will adopt the means by which I have succeeded in becoming young again. At least in my actions there is no indication of physical deterioration, nor is there any suggestion of the gait of an old man. In fact, the activity of all of my actions is always commented on by the various scientific gentlemen who have become interested in my physical condition, and being experts in this direction, their criticism is significant and to me, valuable.

In advanced years, or say at the age of seventy-two, the gait of an old man is usually shuffling and as he walks, the feet are no longer lifted free from the ground. He does not rise upon his toes and the soles of his feet are kept nearly flat; therefore, he drags them cumbersomely and his gait merits the term of shuffling. There is evidently a lessened power in the action of the muscles and a lessened control over them. This is "The Gait of Age," but it does not apply in my case, nor is there any decrease in my elasticity. In proof of which in the presence of several scientific and other interested persons, I ran at the Stadium race track in this city, San Francisco, California, shortly after my seventy-first birthday, one mile in seven minutes and fifty-five seconds (7.55), pulling up at the finish without any distress, and by the time I had leisurely divested myself of my exercising clothes and running shoes, say in about ten minutes, my pulse was beating as steadily as it was when I started. This is ridiculously slow time for a runner, but my action was only that of a steady jog-trot; still any business man, thirty years my junior, will find the distance in the given time rather more of an effort, and not so easy to recover from, than it was in his college days. Furthermore, it would certainly have been impossible for me to accomplish the feat thirty years ago. I do not advise such continued effort after middle age, but was willing to give the exhibition to demonstrate to these gentlemen that my bodily elasticity and endurance were that which might be expected of a man of half of my years. As the pulsation of my heart returned so quickly to normal and the latest clinical report of a very able surgeon is that every organ is in a sound, healthy condition, I believe I am physically in the condition of a healthy young man. As my face is free from wrinkles, the only indication of my age is my gray hair, and from some experiments that I have been making, to which I will refer in the succeeding chapters, I think it may be possible to restore it to its original color, or at least to some extent.

Upon the arterial system, from the largest artery to the smallest capillary, man's physical condition depends. It is evident that the arterial system must be kept free from all clogging matter, for if this is not done, the muscles and organs are not properly supplied with blood or material for repairs and therefore, in that condition, will surely deteriorate and show indications of what we know as age. Such a body cannot be healthy or elastic as it would practically be an old body, and the man or woman in such a condition would be aged even though his or her years were in number those of youth. I am of the opinion that the character of the water we drink has much to do with the sedimentary deposits, and is a factor in producing hardening of the arteries. This seems more than probable, as in countries where the water is strongly charged with lime arteriosclerosis is usually prevalent.

Again quoting from investigations in this direction made by Dr. De Lacy Evans, he says of The Cretins of the Alps, Pyrenees, or other countries where these cases abound: "Lime or magnesian lime is found in excess in the water and while cretinism has two distinct causes, the first and most important cause is the lime or magnesian lime taken into the system, that is, in water used for drinking purposes."

The age of Cretins is short, few of them reach thirty years, and although they die early, they soon present the appearance of age, this miserable state of existence being due to a great extent to premature ossification, the hardening of the arteries. One of the remedies proposed by the scientist is the exclusive use of distilled water. This method is in common use for the prevention of calcareous incrustations in boiler tubes, but with human beings the difficulty of carrying it into general practice with the great mass of humanity, is evident. As a laboratory method or to be practiced only by that exceedingly small minority who can afford to, or to whom it is convenient, it might be partially successful, but it would seem to be as generally difficult to practice as the adoption of a diet of foods carrying the least proportion of lime, which is a plausible theory but not universally practicable.

To become generally in vogue, any method of deferring age by preventing sedimentary deposits in the system, or to any extent eliminating them if they have accrued, must be effective, inexpensive and within the reach of all.

After many years of experimentation in this direction, I can confidently state that the methods of physical rejuvenation which I practice fill those requirements, and as already stated, you will find them clearly described in this book.

The process of cleansing the arteries, whether the largest tube in the system or the most microscopic capillary, can only be accomplished through mechanical means, that is, by the alternate contraction or relaxation of the muscles of the body, that being Nature's method of cleansing it of such debris. It cannot be accomplished by any other means, all medical preparations, however highly recommended, or dietary systems to the contrary. If the arterial system can be kept clear of these deposits, its walls will remain in the elastic condition characteristic of youth, the heart will pump the blood through them without difficulty, while the muscles and organs therefore, being properly nourished, will retain their vigor, and the body may present the appearance of youth, even at an advanced age. We cannot finally defy old age, but its approach can be materially deferred. That this can be accomplished is demonstrated in my own person, for I have been an old man at fifty and now at seventy-two am young again.

Regarding dietetic methods of deferring old age as suggested by the various scientists whom I quote in this and the succeeding chapter, there is another and a very important reason why such systems cannot be as efficacious as these gentlemen claim.

These clogging deposits are not composed wholly of extraneous limey or chalky matter, such as Dr. Evans has described, for in the process of life, worn-out tissues or dead cells result. This debris, or ashes, is the result of that process, and a great proportion of it remains in the system, clogging up its various organs and impeding their functions. Therefore, if this debris is not eliminated, old age cannot be satisfactorily deferred, nor can life be materially prolonged. And neither food systems nor medicinal preparations can rectify the conditions. The remedy lies in Nature's method, muscular activity. There is no other effectual means by which such debris can be removed. Diet as you will, stuff yourself with health foods, saturate your system with the most widely advertised medicine preparations for the attainment of health, strength, activity and longevity, you will not succeed by one or all of such means. It has never been accomplished by any lymph, serum, elixir or medicine yet brought before the world, and when the human structure is carefully studied it does not seem that it ever will be. I repeat my assertion that the only successful eliminative process is Nature's method, which is muscular activity; that is, mechanically forcing such clogging matter out of the system by the alternate contraction and relaxation of every muscle of the body. That is the secret of physical rejuvenation.

In the almost unceasing activity of childhood and early youth, we see the manifestation of Nature's method of removing dead matter from our bodies. The restless action of a caged animal is but another instance of the same method. In all ages, man has vainly endeavored to restore to the aged human body by medicinal means, the elasticity and vitality characteristic of youth. This was the disappointed dream of the early alchemist, it is even now the faint, half-hearted hope of Science; but as years roll on, bearing with them the precedent of countless millions of failures, and not one authenticated success, that hope is becoming more dim, the doubt increasing. Still we struggle on upon the same misleading, beaten track, but before the end of this century I predict that the simple but effectual methods for the prevention of age and prolongation of life which I practice will very largely take the place of medicinal methods in the treatment of aged persons, and that physical culture methods generally will be considered of the first importance in the science of gerocomy.

To know how to keep physically young, you should know why you grow old. The human anatomy is composed of millions of minute microscopical bodies which science terms cells. These cells come into being through the air you breathe, the liquid you drink, and the food you eat, and then by the marvelous process of digestion and assimilation are converted into cellular tissue. Having come into being, these minute cells live their brief life and then die just as you and I must die, and having become dead matter must be eliminated from the system. If not, they clog up the body and impede its functions. Under these circumstances it rapidly deteriorates, the muscles not being properly nourished, shrink and the signs of age appear. If this clogging waste matter can be eliminated, then the conditions of youth will return. This can never be accomplished by medicinal means, Nature alone provides the method. It lies, as I have stated, in the alternate contraction and relaxation of the muscles. In that way you force out from the body any waste matter which may have deposited into the venous and glandular system, and it is then carried off by the ordinary bodily excretions. Any muscle or set of muscles so exercised will increase in size, strength and elasticity, and will finally be practically rejuvenated. This being true of one muscle, it is true of all and as all parts of the body are in sympathy with each other, any adjacent gland or organ will be benefited. Therefore, if all parts of the structure are so exercised a general rejuvenation results. My method is simply the using of a systematic series of contractions and alternate relaxations of every large muscle or sets of muscles of the body. These exercises I practice while lying in bed, comfortably ensconced under the bedclothes. By this means and the other simple methods I describe, I have accomplished my rejuvenation. These movements might be described as a kind of muscle-pumping process, as that is what exercise really is, if health alone is your object, for mechanical appliances are not necessary. This system is especially adapted for those in advanced years or of sedentary modes of life, and is equally beneficial and advisable for either sex. The exercises that commence at page 91 are illustrated by thirty photographs taken from life. You will find them easily learned and remarkably effective. This is a certain means of throwing off dead matter which, as I have repeatedly stated, is the principal cause of old age. In my case rheumatism, dyspepsia and other minor ailments have departed long ago, and at seventy-two there is no longer any evidence of physical deterioration.

But in considering the causes of old age there is also another and a very important factor to be taken into consideration and that is the condition of the glandular function. In old age there is usually inactivity in this direction, defective assimilation being therefore a marked characteristic of advanced years. With that condition there is a loss in flesh and while it exists, it is impossible to build up the body. The remedy lies in general muscular activity. This, if practiced with all of the muscles of the body, will mechanically stimulate all glandular action, and whether that function is of the nature of secretion or excretion, greater activity will follow and the result will be improved assimilation, and as that function is the basis of life, it is evident that health will be therefore improved. This is all very simple and logical when it is explained, but the fact that the secret of healthy glandular action lay in the mechanical process of adjacent muscular activity was, for a long time, a difficult crux to me. Naturally, you think that I could find the explanation in any work upon health methods or physiology, but you are mistaken. At least, no especial significance seems to have been attached to this vitally important fact. Reliable books clearly describing proven methods of deferring old age are very scarce, and I have usually been compelled to solve the problems myself, for I have been prospecting a route to health and longevity, seemingly little considered and never travelled to any considerable extent by any one. I also regret to say that, after carefully reading the best known books dealing with the subject, I came to the conclusion that their authors were a kind of scientific, literary cuttlefish, who by discharging a cloud of ink and an unnecessary amount of scientific terms, obscured the subject and added but little information to it. The trouble principally being that with the exception of Lewis Cornaro, to whose book I will later refer, they wrote of the experiences of others but never of their own. My confidence in the efficacy of the methods I advise are the results of my own personal, successful experience with them.

One of the problems that once badly puzzled me was, that I found that very thin people often gained flesh by these exercises, while those suffering from a surplus of adipose tissue lost that unwelcome superfluity. In the former case, the explanation is found in the stimulation of the glandular action as described; therefore, improved assimilation brings an increase of flesh, and more healthful conditions, while with the stout persons muscular activity worked off the unwholesome superfluous fat.

There seems to be a certain physical standard or outline, which is ours at birth and by heritage, and the nearer we approach that outline, the healthier we will be. Health is really the condition of equilibrium, between assimilation and elimination, and if reached the result is perfect health.

Nature's plan is, that we should all reach and maintain that condition; why so few of us do so is our own fault. If assimilation and elimination are in perfect equilibrium and the mind is as healthfully active as the body, then you have reached the condition which Nature intended and will warrant the expectation of your living to the full limit of the term fixed for your stay here, which is one hundred years. But to accomplish this, your mental attitude must also be considered and this is a very important matter, for undoubtedly a mental activity and a hopeful, cheerful disposition are great factors in the prolongation of life, and just as certainly the contrary attitude will shorten it. If your general impression is "that the world is liable to fall off and break in two," that "fate has it in for you," that you were "born to hard luck," that you "never had a chance and never will have one," and that "you will not live long anyway," then, of course, you will lose courage and without the will to spur you on to effort, you will not succeed either in your business or in prolonging your life. That pessimistic state of mind retards your digestion and has a bad effect upon your liver. Such despondent people are usually unhealthy and therefore unhappy, feeling that "there is nothing to live for" they usually age more rapidly than optimistic people. The remedy lies in both physical and mental activity, for the same law applies to the mental organization as to the rest of your body, so that if you would keep young mentally you must exercise your brains. The list of old men, thinkers, writers, statesmen and orators, who have achieved their greatest successes in advanced years, is too long to recite, but the secret of their success in every case was, that they kept busy.

There is an old German proverb, "If you rest you rust." It is true, and if you would be healthy and prolong your life, don't get into a rusty condition, either mentally or physically. If you do, then, like any other piece of machinery, your term of usefulness being past, you will be relegated to the junk pile and your stay here will be shortened. There is a close sympathy between the mind and the body and if either deteriorates the other will speedily share in its deterioration. Therefore, keep active mentally as well as physically, and the easiest and most effective method of keeping your body active and therefore healthy, will be found fully described in the book.

But as to exercising your brains, that is a matter which depends largely upon your tastes, habits, environments and natural abilities. Have an interest in human affairs. If you are a woman, in your leisure hours take an interest in church matters, charities, settlement work, club affairs, in short, any wholesome amusement to keep you busy and occupy your mind. Society should also engage your attention if your tastes run that way and environments permit. But as Shakespeare says, "Society is no comfort to one not sociable." If so, then become a member of some religious organization and go to church. While I do not belong to any sect, and have a religion of my own, yet I have a high respect for churches and church people, for I have realized after many years' experience as a choir singer in various churches, that there I found the best people, and such people will be of value to you and make life more pleasant.

But don't join any church where the "Terrors of the Lord," and the awful fate which befall those who don't agree with such ideas are preached. If you do your dyspepsia will be worse and you won't be happy. I speak from experience, as my people were Presbyterians of the ultra-puritan type and I was brought up on the "Shorter Catechism," "Infant Damnation," and the "Fires of Hell." This spiritual Sunday diet, in combination with cold mince pie and fried doughnuts, laid the foundation of the digestive disorders which troubled me for many years afterwards. Moral: If you have any tendencies to dyspepsia or suicidal melancholy, don't join that kind of a church. But hunt up something modern and progressive, some church where you will meet cheerful people, people who have made their church popular by the social amusements possible to such a congregation. And if the leader of that congregation, whether clergyman, priest or Rabbi, is a believer in sunshine, fresh air and out-of-doors pleasure, that is the church to belong to, for there you will find the kind of society which will assist you in maintaining a cheerful disposition, be an aid to health and one of the factors in deferring old age.

The Will in Exercising

THE effect of the will upon the body is very marked in these exercises. Each set of muscles being exercised by itself, there is a concentration of thought, or determination of will force, to that point and it would seem that the speedy and very remarkable muscular development often resulting from the practice of this muscle-tensing system is due as much to the will force concentrated upon the muscles placed in action as by the exercises. On first thought this statement may not find favor with the average reader, but when you consider some of the phenomena which are undoubtedly caused by the action of the will this theory of the cause of the rapid muscular growth is not illogical.

I quote at random from a number of medical authorities:

"By force of will the beating of the heart may become slower or quicker or may even cease under the stress of emotions, such as anger or fear."

"A very great fright may even cause death or syncope."

"Concentrated attention, that is, attention

concentrated on any portion of our body, produces manifest changes there; thus, redness or paleness may be induced in the face or swellings on different parts of the body."

"Certain monks are known to have induced the red marks of flagellation or the signs of Christ's sufferings upon their bodies, and it is an established fact that by fixing the attention upon any part of the body positive pains may be produced."

"Rage affects the salivary glands."

"Fear disturbs the functions of the heart and anxiety the digestive organs."

It is evident, therefore, in view of the phenomena instanced, that the will has much to do with the determination of our lives and our physical conformation, impressing our character and modes of thought upon our features, and in exercise, and especially in these muscle-tensing exercises, it is a very important factor in muscular development. The will also has a law in common with the muscular system, that is, it grows in strength when exercised.

If things were always as hard to do as when tried for the first time we would never progress, but the way becomes easier as we continue our efforts and exercise the will, so that those who practice these exercises will find the desire to execute them grow, the difficulties first encountered disappear and finally that which was distasteful becomes an attractive habit.

Mentality has much to do with our health and the duration of our lives. A fixed determination to live will prolong life just as certainly as the feeling that we are growing old lessens our courage and hastens the end. If we lose faith in our strength it leaves us. If we believe that age is beginning to weigh heavily upon us we take to sedentary habits and little by little we lapse into sluggish lives, our blood is vitiated by idleness, our feebly renewed tissues and lowered vitality invite diseases which we know as the signs of age. We lose courage and faith in ourselves and then truly become old.

It is a worn but truthful adage that "every one is as old as he thinks himself to be." If you think yourself aging, surely you will hasten that condition and marks of physical decay appear which your years may not warrant. Moral: Don't admit to yourself, or to any other person, that you are growing old, and if you resolutely deny the approach of indications of age you will retard their appearance.

Remember this: When you think young and act young, people think you are a good deal younger than you are and finally you will come to believe it yourself. When you have reached that stage you will have the courage of your convictions and the battle is half won. You will have pride in your physical improvement and, fearing physical deterioration, you will try to keep trying and success will surely come to you.

An example of the power of the will over the body is found in faith cure, or Christian Science, as beyond all question great numbers of well authenticated cures of dangerous diseases have been effected, amply demonstrating its efficiency, but these cures are due to a settled conviction of the efficacy of the method and not to theology, being simply a demonstration of the power of the mind over the body and a verification of the statement that the thought of any given bodily change tends to the actual production of the change that thought suggests. Hence the success of mental or faith cure.

It is a well-demonstrated fact that a disease can be induced by brooding over it, so it can in many cases be cured by believing that it does not exist, that being the basis of Christian Science. A fixed determination to be well and implicit faith in a remedy or formula, however fantastic and illogical from a scientific standpoint, bringing about the results desired, though all scientific reasons why it cannot be so should be to the contrary.

The world in all ages has been full of records of innumerable instances of healing through the power of the mind. Science gives no philosophical explanation but simply dumps the records upon the ash heap of superstition and yet for hundreds of years the "King's touch" was a sovereign remedy for scrofula and cured it in innumerable instances. And at this day thousands of well-authenticated cures of serious diseases and of instances of the removal of physical deformities which have baffled surgery and the medical profession remain to the credit of the various methods of mental healing. Why? Because the will is the directing power of the mechanism of your body, and when you have obtained control of that power you are close in touch with the great principle of life —the mystery no man yet has solved, and whose limit science cannot determine. But there must be a method, a system of will control, or concentration of thought, to effect the object desired.

In Christian Science that method can be found in "Science and Health," by Mrs. Eddy. This book for the most part is simply a collection of religious quotations, lacking both scientific reasons and logic, but the effect of the faithful reading and contemplation of the various marvelous cures instanced seems to have a tendency to place the mind in a receptive condition favorable to suggestion. The disjointed religious sentences, the iteration and reiteration of the ideas, "There is no disease," "Have faith," "You are not sick," "You are well," "You are cured," will finally carry conviction, and if the reader is of the faith and has the confidence which its teachings demand, the chances are that he will actually be cured. And so of these exercises. If you can understand that with every muscular contraction and its alternate relaxation you are expelling the worn-out and dead tissue which is the real cause of physical age, you will be encouraged to go on, and as you do so and you find your physical condition and health improving, confidence in yourself, faith in the system I describe, will come to you and success in your efforts will surely be yours.

To concentrate attention upon the muscles you are endeavoring to develop, count the movements and try to remember the position as shown in the illustration of the exercise you are practicing.

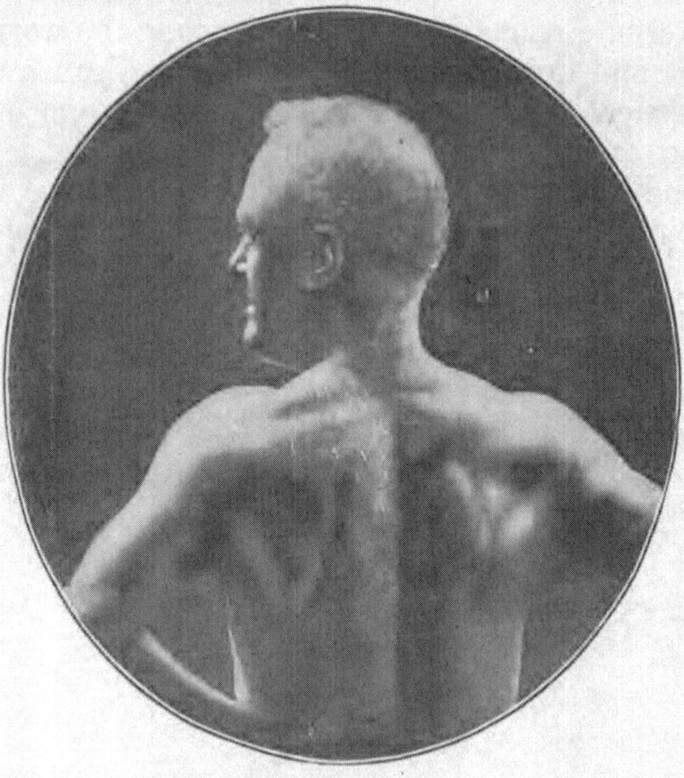

Result of Exercising the Muscles of the Back at 72

Exercising in Bed

IF you have read and carefully considered the matter elsewhere presented in this book, you will realize that the secret of my health, elasticity of body and unprecedented return to the condition of physical youth at my advanced age are principally due to the persistent practice of the series of muscular contractions and alternate relaxations, which I describe under the title of "Exercising in Bed." And as I do not differ from other human beings in my physical structure, what has been possible in my case is just as possible in yours. Bear this always in mind—all muscles and all organs grow in size, strength and elasticity if properly exercised, and they all surely lose those properties if this is neglected. In short, the secret of my methods of getting young, keeping young and possessing the bodily elasticity of youth, lies principally in systematic and persistent muscular activity. Strict attention must, of course, be paid to cleanliness, both internal and external; also the food eaten must be properly prepared for digestion by chewing it thoroughly before it is swallowed. But if exercise is not a part of your system of health, success is doubtful. I have heretofore given in detail the reasons why we grow old and why general muscular activity will eliminate the sedimentary deposits, which are principally the cause of old age, and why the form of exercise I practice is of such marked benefit to both the glandular structure and circulating system. But if you do not clearly understand me, I would suggest that you read those chapters over again, as I believe I can add no further information which would assist you in your prospective experiments.

That is in the art of getting physically young again. If you neglect to exercise, and in that way expel the clogging ashes of the system, due to the process of life, your body will surely stiffen and become rusty, just like any other piece of machinery. Then you cannot be healthy. Your usefulness will be impaired and you will show marks of age.

Systematic, persistent and general muscular activity will expel that rust or clogging debris, and then you will commence to "limber up." And if the various simple health methods I advise are faithfully practiced, you may again become "just as good as new." No, not altogether. I must admit that it is not possible to make a very young body—by this or any other health system—out of a very old one, but the improvement will soon be so considerable as to be a source of great satisfaction to you.

Also you will stay here very much longer than if your machine was in a rusty, clogged-up state. For that is the condition of old age. You will probably admit the truth of what I say; unless you are hopelessly a believer in attempting to secure health by drug methods.

But you may be under the impression that to obtain the benefit of exercise you must join a gymnasium or perform a variety of violent motions at unpleasant hours, and possibly, with inconvenient surroundings. Also you will think you will need a physical culture instructor. Ordinarily, yes, but in this system you will need no teacher, other than the instructions here presented.

The thirty exercises described and illustrated in this chapter are all performed while lying in bed, and as each set of exercises is very simple, you will have no difficulty in learning them. Each set of muscles is brought into activity by itself, and as all of the movements are executed slowly, the bed-clothes need not be disarranged, while if your movements are deliberate, neither will the pulse be unduly accelerated.

This last is very important, as in gymnasium work, over-exertion greatly accelerates the pulse and a consequent strain upon the heart often results. This is very injurious, as enlargement of the heart is a serious matter.

The running path, bars, punching bag and the

various other appliances of a well-appointed gymnasium cannot be too highly recommended, as they form an excellent road to health, also a good method of obtaining strength and elasticity of body. But it is very possible to overdo the matter. Therefore be careful. It is not possible to successfully prepare the body for an athletic event demanding great exertion without the use of such adjuncts and regular training, but as a preliminary to getting into regular condition any athlete will find these muscle-tensing exercises, performed while lying in bed, will very materially lessen the time usually required to get into first-class condition.

To do this, instead of the few movements allotted to the exercises described as necessary to health, simply increase them, and you can work up every muscle of your body and reduce fat. But the first time you try the movements sharp and fast you will get so tired that you will not feel like boxing, doing road work or anything else of a strenuous nature next day.

It is the same thing as gymnasium work without the appliances, but I write simply for those advanced in years or sedentary people, those whose only aim is health. And such people should confine themselves to the few movements I advise for each set of muscles. Don't try to learn and practice them all at once. Go slow and learn each set by itself before you take up the next.

There is still another advantage of my system as compared with gymnasium practice. In the "gym" one is very likely to develop one set of muscles and neglect others that are equally important. The body, therefore, gets out of balance and like any other badly-balanced machinery, is not capable of the efficiency Nature has intended that it should have. But in the system of exercise I am describing, all of the muscles are brought into activity, and a generally even development results. In my case I am evenly developed all over, a fact that has always been specially commented upon by those surgeons who have examined me.

An objection to exercise as a health method is the way that it encroaches on one's time. Under the usual hurried conditions of modern life this is often true, although your health is far more important than your business. But with this system of exercise, this need not be an objection. In my own case I practice the exercises at a time when I am absolutely idle, that is, I habitually wake at about 5:30 A.M. I do not rise, but leisurely commence the movements, one after the other, and during the next half hour, or more, I practice them all.

By that time I have systematically brought into action every muscle of my body. A healthy glow and a wide-awake feeling and ready for business have resulted. The windows are wide open; the air is pure; the bed warm and comfortable, and the sun is probably streaming in with its life-giving rays. I have been exercising continuously but slowly for over half an hour. My heart is beating steadily. Then I get up, shave, take a quick tepid bath all over, and being perfectly healthy, I realize the joy of living to the full!

If you have the blues, if your liver is torpid and you have a dark-brown taste in your mouth don't "take something for it," that is, don't take any medicines. Try my plan and you will not regret it.

If you faithfully follow my instructions, the chances are ten to one that the result will be health, elasticity of body and a prolongation of your life. These are the greatest and truest of riches that the world can offer you and when you have them you wouldn't exchange them for the assets of the Bank of England with a colony of billionaires thrown in for good measure!

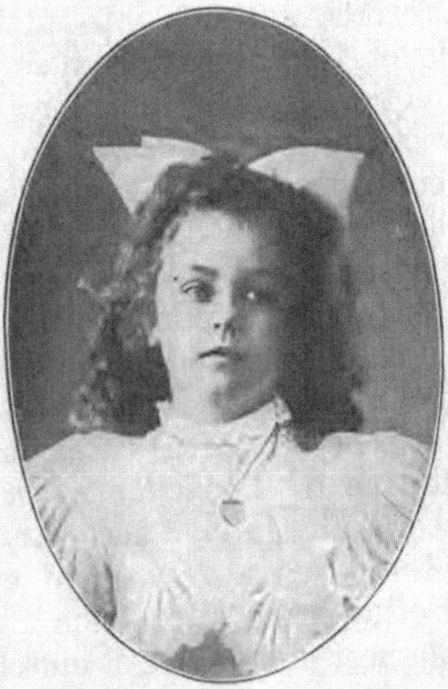

A Young but Very Successful Disciple of This System of Physical Culture

Thirty Exercises

THESE exercises bring into action every muscle of the human body. They are all practiced while lying in bed, and under cover of the bed-clothes.

The number of movements advisable for each exercise is designated in figures upon each of the illustrations. If any are not clear, refer to the numbered pages, upon which you will find larger illustrations and more explicit descriptions of the exercises. Do not try to learn too many at once. Learn each one before taking up the next. The changes in position may not seem absolutely necessary, but I have found that even a very slight change of position will often bring into action an entirely new set of muscles; sometimes of muscles which do not seem to be a part of that action. Therefore, if you desire general muscular activity, which is the key-note of this system, do not omit these slight changes in positions, and do not execute the movements too quickly. Nothing is gained by rapid action, as this surely results in acceleration of the pulse, which is not advisable; the object is to stimulate circulation and healthy glandular activity, but not to overdo it. A steady, deliberate rate of action will be found far more beneficial, and then no evil results will follow, as, under those conditions, no stress is placed upon the heart.

Do not flounce around in bed as you practice the movements; you will only disarrange the bed-clothes. That is not necessary, and if the movements are performed with deliberation it will not happen. My experience has been that most people commence this or any other system of physical culture by going too fast. As a consequence, they soon become sore, discouraged, and give it up. Don't fall into that error. Learn this system just as you would learn typewriting or the piano; *i. e.*, one thing at a time, and when you can execute a number of these movements without getting confused, you will be surprised to find how easy it all is and how rapidly you improve in health.

At the risk of being charged with egotism, I will say that it is not advisable for you to try to devise any new movements in this direction, because I have been experimenting upon all of the muscles of my body for over twenty years, and whatever new exercises of this nature you may think you have devised, I have tried them long before you did, and there is some good reason for their omission from the list presented. This is a strong statement, but after over twenty years' study of the "pulls" of the various muscles of my body, I think you will find that the ground has been thoroughly covered, and only those movements have been retained which are of absolute necessity in this "lazy man's system of exercise." I will modify that statement, at least as to three of the exercises described, in which mechanical appliances are used. For the purposes of health alone I do not believe those appliances are necessary; *i. e.*, for general muscular activity they are included in the list. Not because I now use them, but because many people think they are necessary, and still use them with excellent results.

It is true that the mechanical appliances of a well-appointed gymnasium are necessary to prepare the body for any athletic feats, but as the object of this book is simply to show sedentary people, or old people like myself, the way to physical rejuvenation, I advise you to follow my directions, and not waste your time in trying to devise new muscular movements not necessary in your case. You will find all you require in the list presented. I am often asked if I approve of running as an exercise. Certainly, but after you are past boyhood or early manhood, better not exceed a steady jog trot. I always run at that gait two-thirds of a mile every day; that is, one-third in the morning and one-third in the afternoon or evening. This keeps my wind in excellent condition, and I think helps my singing voice. It certainly helps me to maintain my speed, as I can, if need be, run one hundred yards in fifteen seconds, and this without very marked distress. But I wouldn't do it again unless some very urgent reason, like a policeman, was the incentive. And if I were the physical instructor of a lot of youngsters in any college I would discourage the "one-hundred-yard dash," and especially the persistent fast work preparatory to it. In that work too much stress is placed upon the heart, and I have found more cripples in the fast class than in the slower distance runners.

Regarding the two-hundred-and-twenty-yard sprinters up on their toes, every muscle of their bodies at extreme tension, hearts throbbing as if they would burst, eyes fixed, and the do-or-die look of the fast runner at the finish, I can only say, "Don't"; that is, unless such an athlete is a member of the college suicide club, and anxious to obtain a becoming halo and a complimentary epitaph early in life. If so, keep at it; it is then only a question of time. As to walking as an exercise, certainly, and you cannot very well hurt yourself, but always remember that there are no vital organs in the legs. They are only the running gear of the machine. Better endeavor to develop the upper part of the body, as there the muscular structure encases the vital machinery within, and when that muscular structure is strengthened by exercise, those internal organs share in the improvement. Therefore health. I can give you no better advice than to learn and persistently practice the exercises described, then you will be healthy. You can't help it; *i. e.*, if you will follow my advice and the general methods I practice. I will add an excellent exercise for developing the calves of the legs which can easily be practiced, and is very effective. As you lie upon your side, drop the heel as low as possible and then kick downward, say 15 times to commence with. It is not included in the illustrated list of the 30 exercises, as the action could not be clearly shown in the photograph. Repeat upon both sides of the body.

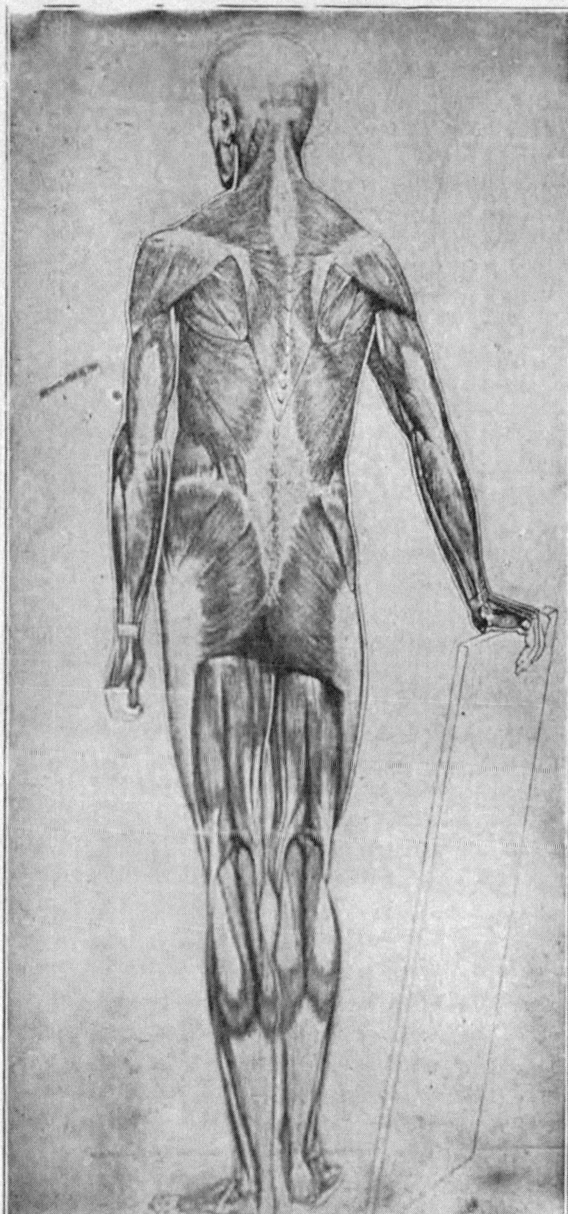

Back View of the Muscles of the Human Body

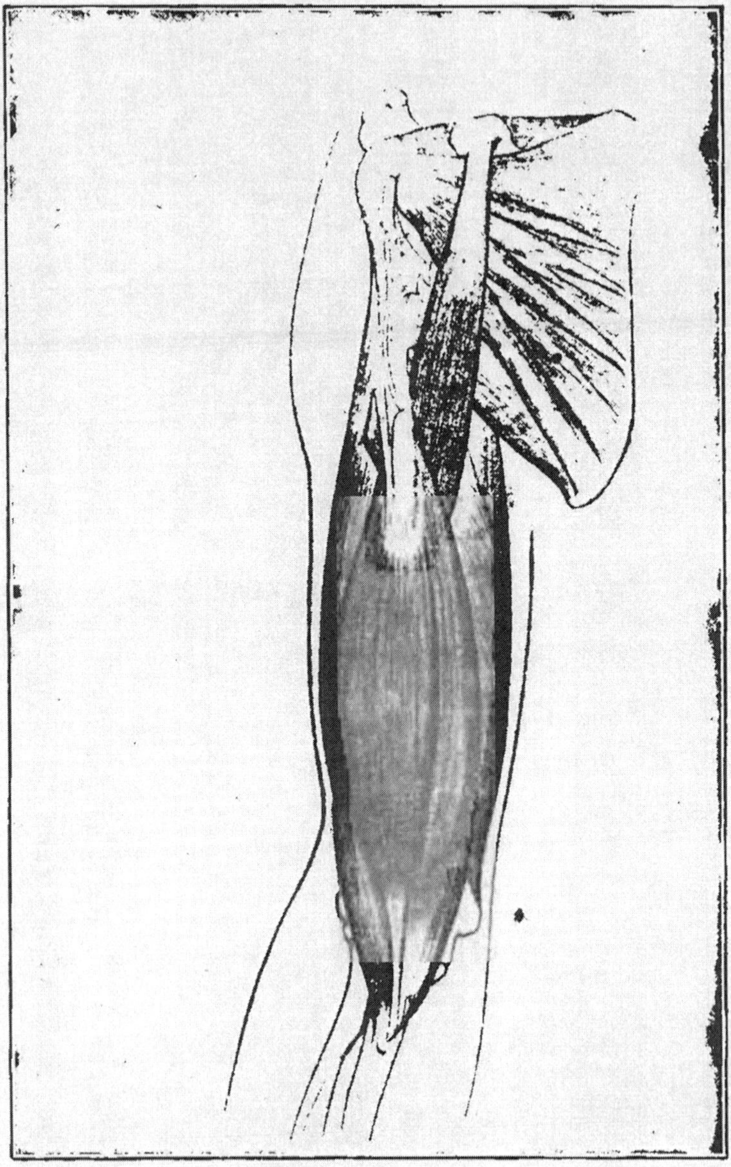

Showing Muscles of the Upper Arm—Side View

Things to Be Remembered

ALL of these exercises are performed in bed under cover of the bed-clothes.

Commence the exercises as soon as you are awake.

Count the movements; this concentrates your attention and growth is then more rapid.

During these exercises frequently take deep breaths.

Keep your windows open both top and bottom.

Breathe through the nose—not the mouth.

Take a tepid plunge bath every morning after exercising; in and out quick.

Learn and practice each exercise before taking up a new one.

Copious water drinking, and especially a glass about fifteen minutes before breakfast, is a remedy for constipation.

Digestion is retarded and digestive organs impaired if you hurry at your meals. Eat slowly and masticate your food thoroughly.

Attend to the calls of Nature promptly.

The chapter upon internal cleanliness, page 168, is important; study it and learn why—it may save your life.

Keep in the sunlight as much as possible.

If you think you are threatened with appendicitis, wash out the lower bowel, the colon (see page 168), and starve—it is more effective than an operation and cheaper.

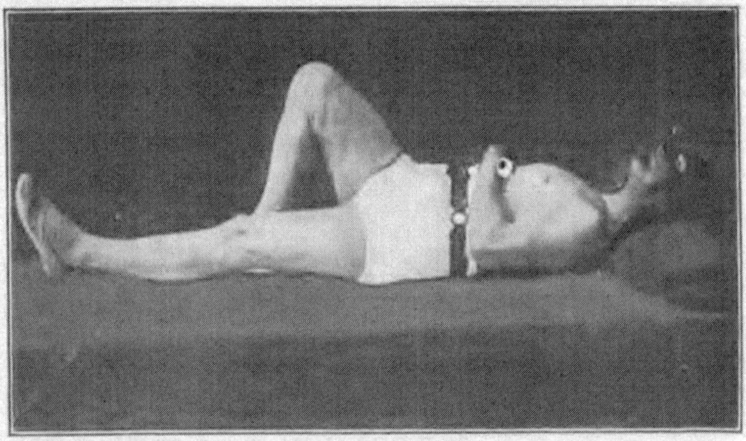

See Page 350. Nos. 1 and 2. The Lower Abdominal Muscles. 5 Movements Alternately

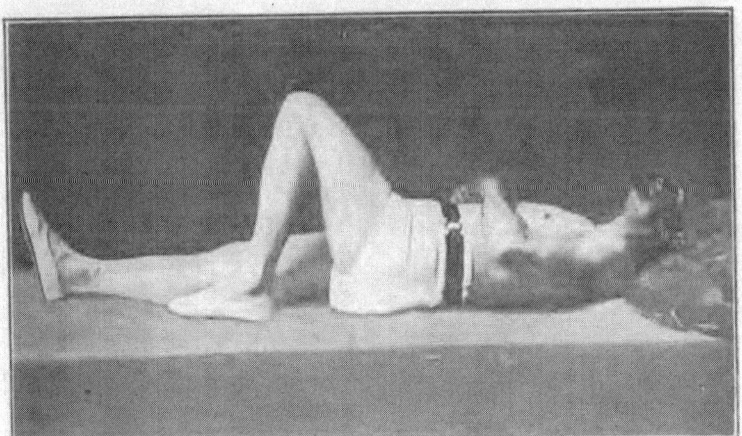

See Page 350. Nos. 1 and 2. Alternately 5 Movements. The Lower Abdominal Muscles

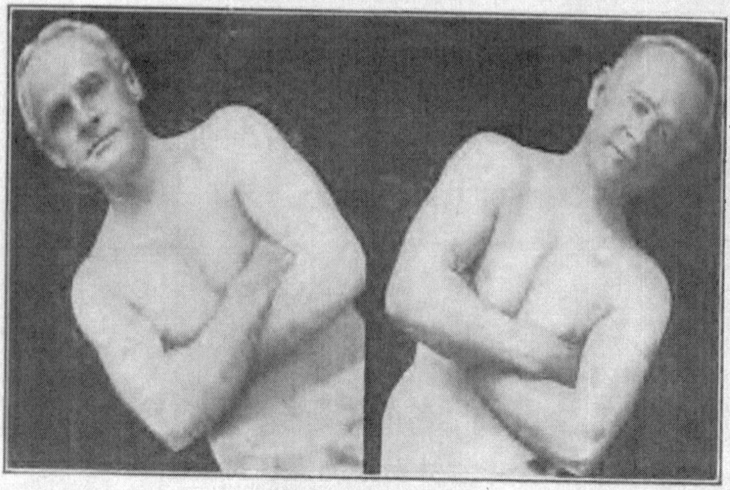

See Page 346. No. 3. Loin Muscles. 5 Movements Alternately

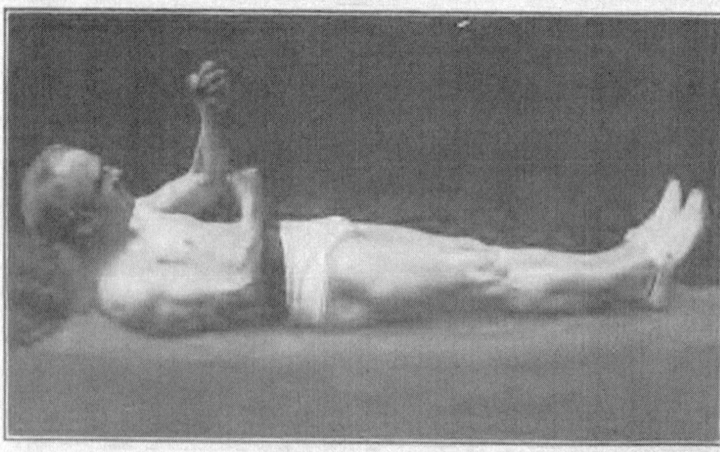

See Page 373. No. 4. Percussion Abdominal Muscles. 5 Movements

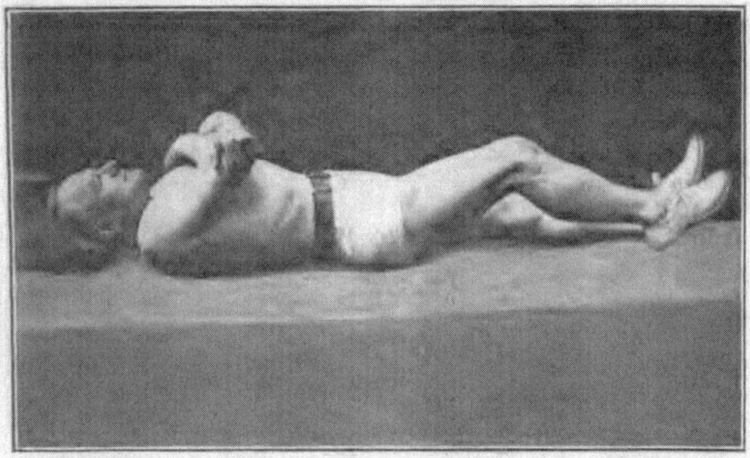

See Page 335. No. 5. Shoulder Shrugging Exercise. 5 Movements

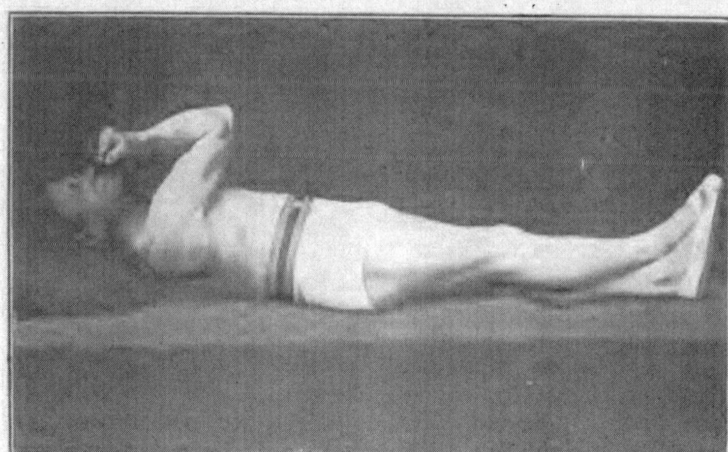

See Page 313. No. 6. Shoulder Blade Muscles. 5 Movements on Each Side

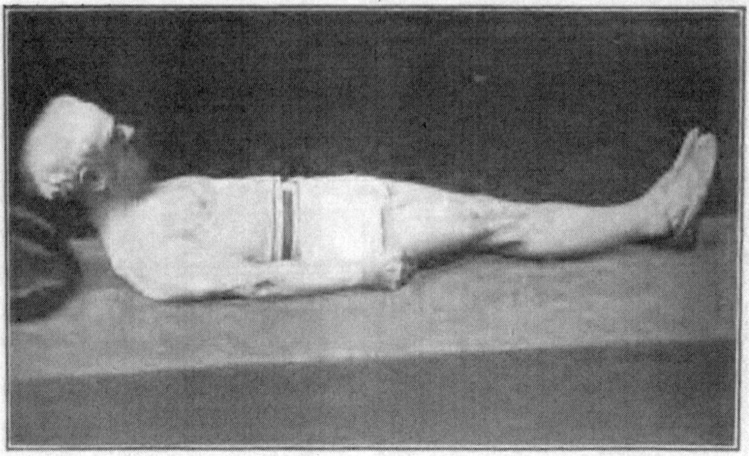

See Page 305. No. 7. Muscles of the Neck and Abdomen. 10 Movements

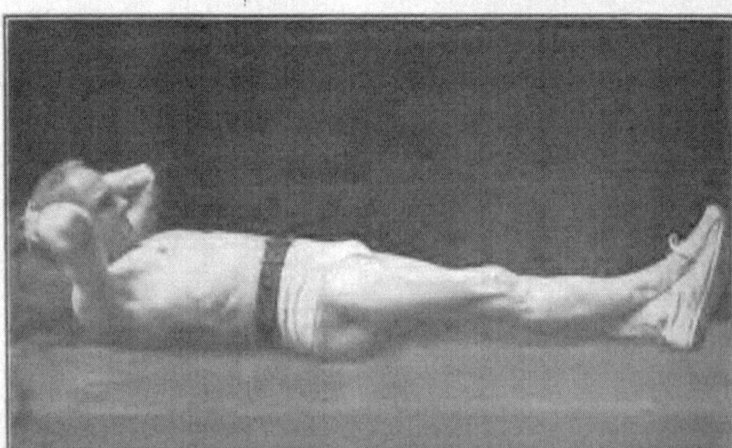

See Page 320. No. 8. Resistance Exercise for Back of Neck. 5 Movements

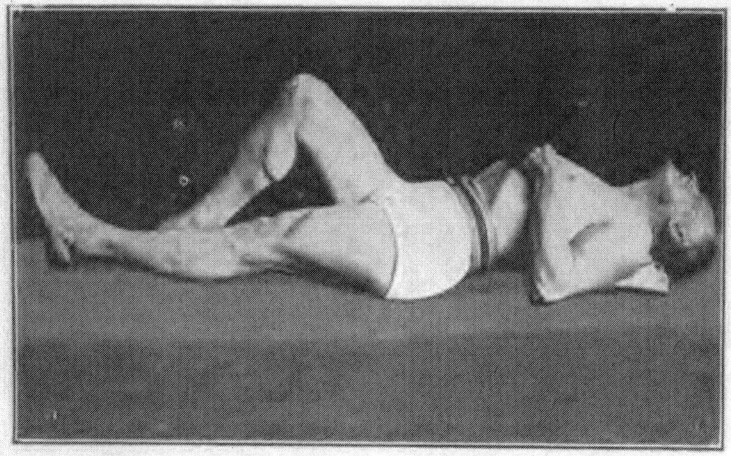

See Page 295. No. 9. Muscles of the Throat. 10 Movements

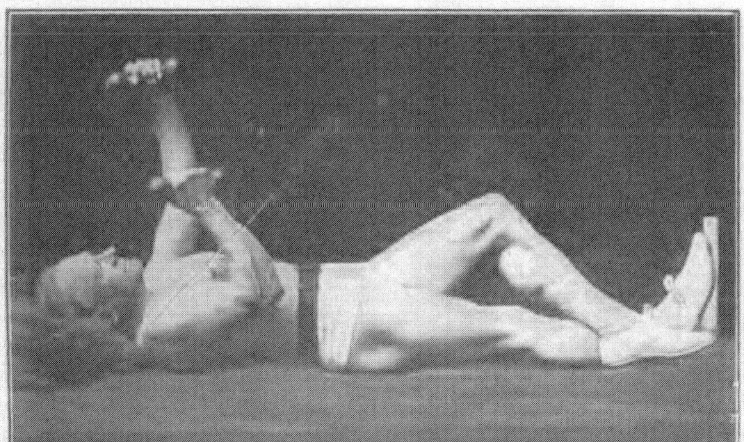

See Page 325. No. 10. Striking Exercise Either With or Without Dumb-bells

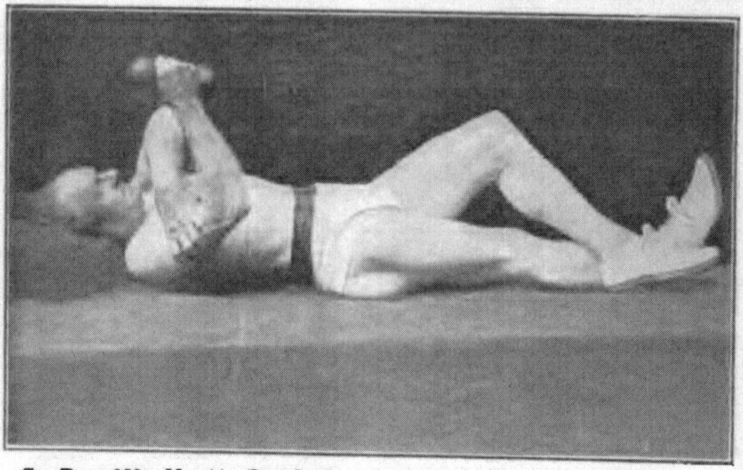

See Page 329. No. 11. Developing the Arms by Dumb-bell Movements with Massage

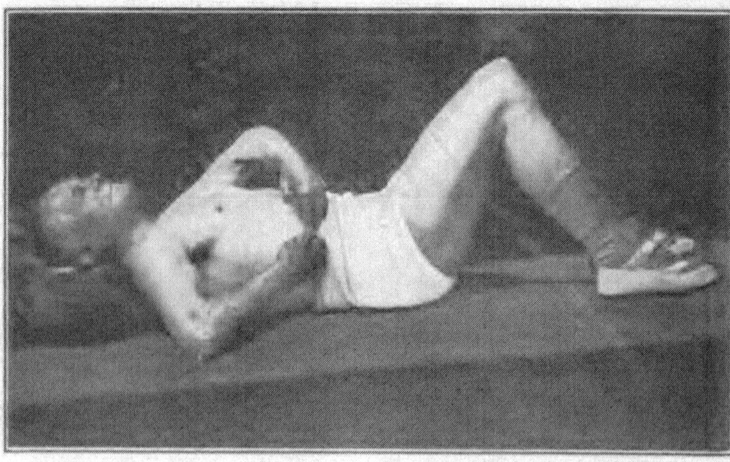

See Page 157. No. 12. Massage of Liver Lying on Back. 10 Movements

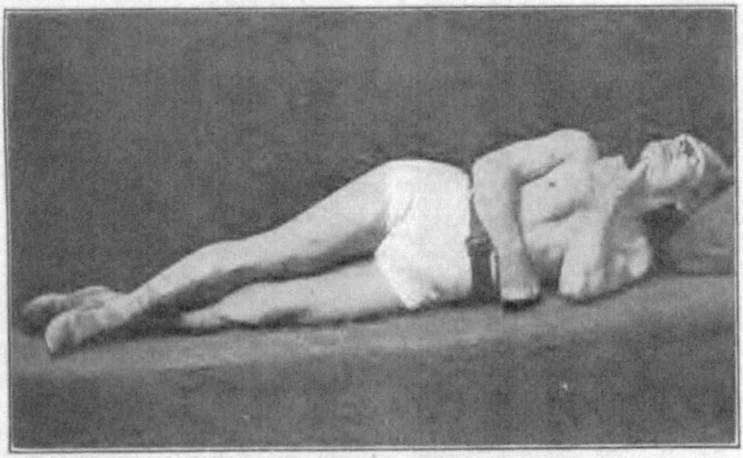

See Page 315. No. 13. Development of the Throat Muscles. 10 Movements

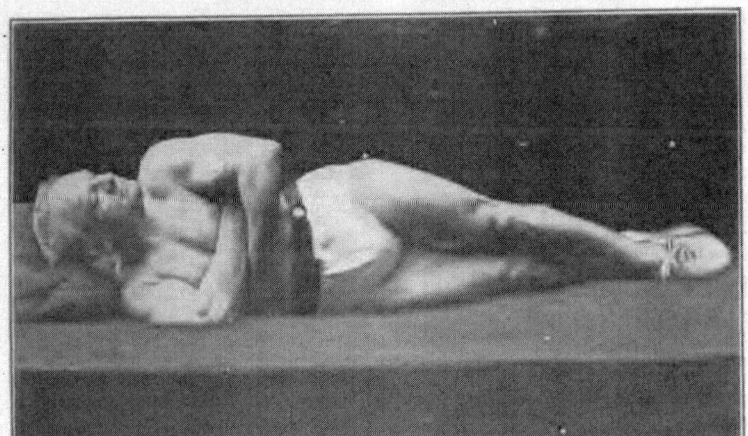

See Page 322. No. 14. Development of the Throat and Neck Muscles. 10 Movements

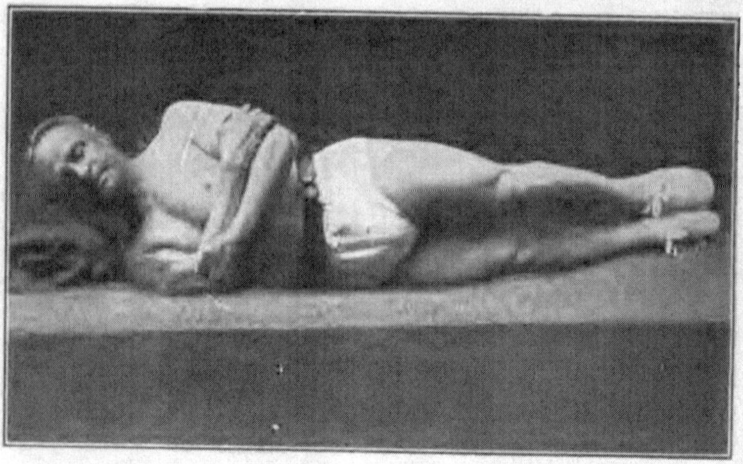

See Page 355. No. 15. Tensing Exercise for the Whole Body.
3 Movements

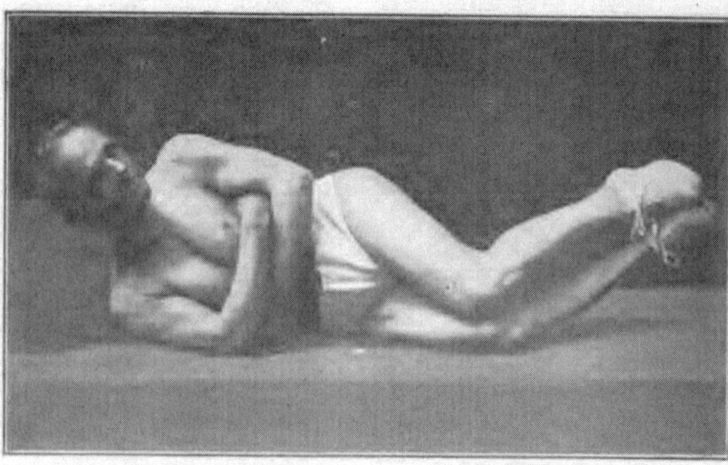

See Page 353. No. 16. Muscles of the Sides. 10 Movements

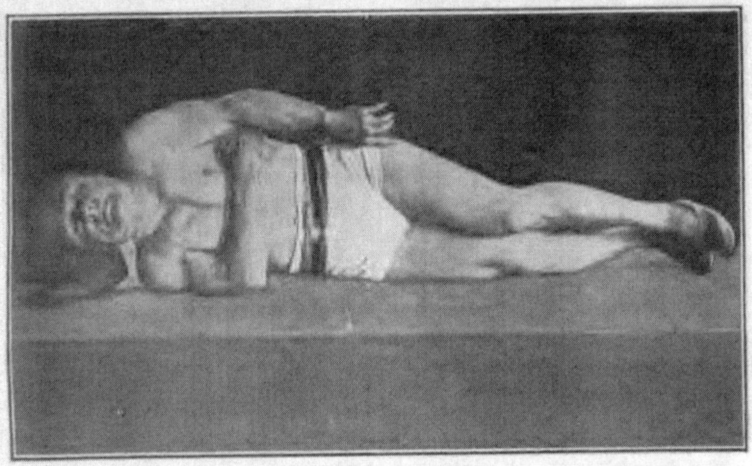

See Page 337. No. 17. Muscles Covering the Shoulder Blades.
5 Movements.

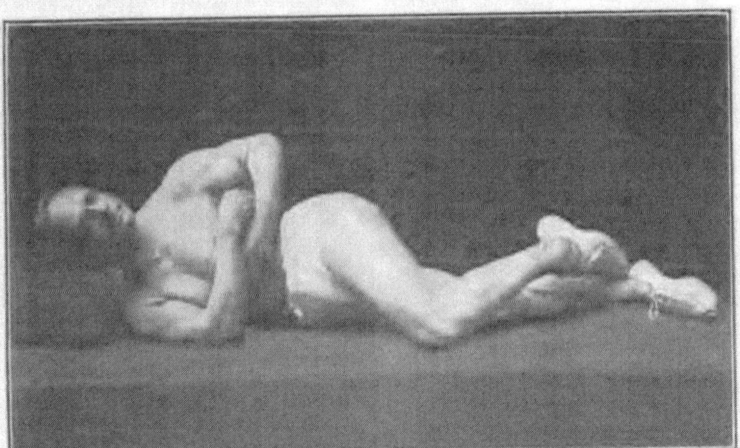

See Page 371. No. 18. Hip and Loins. 5 Movements.

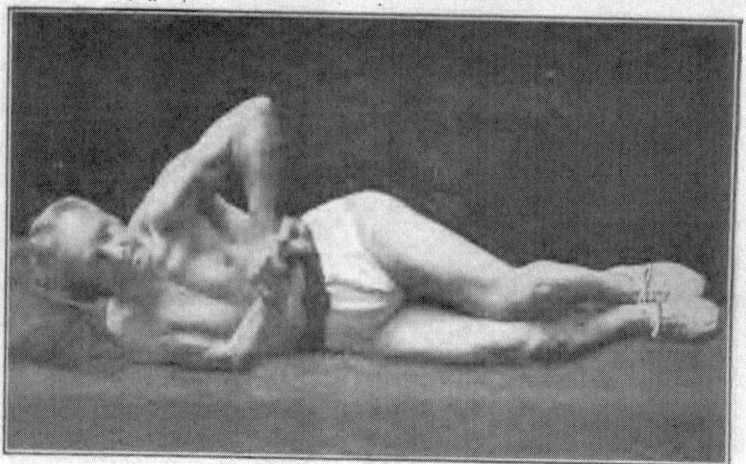

See Page 363. No. 19. Resistance Fore Arm Exercise. 5 Movements

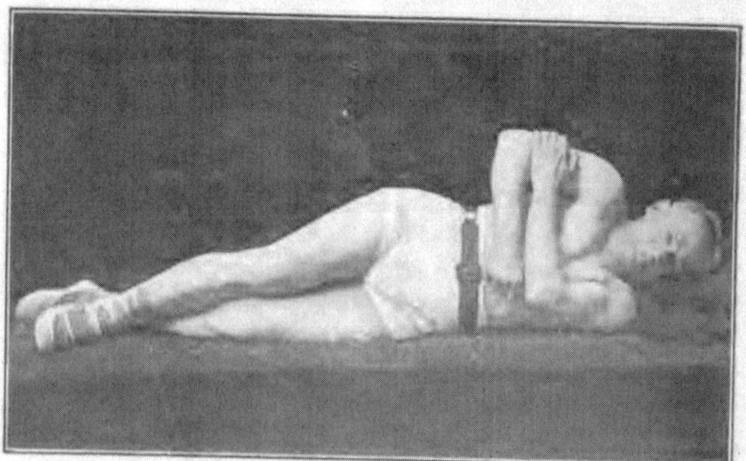

See Page 369. No. 20. Resistance Triceps or Back Muscles of the Arms

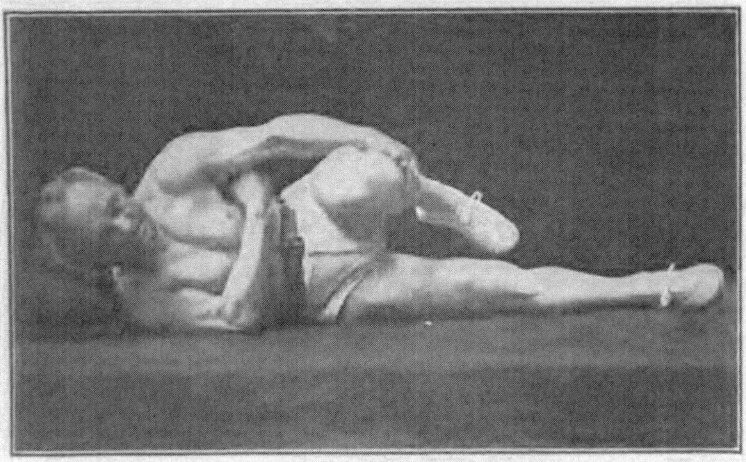

See Page 358. No. 21. Single Arm Pulling Exercise for Shoulder and Back

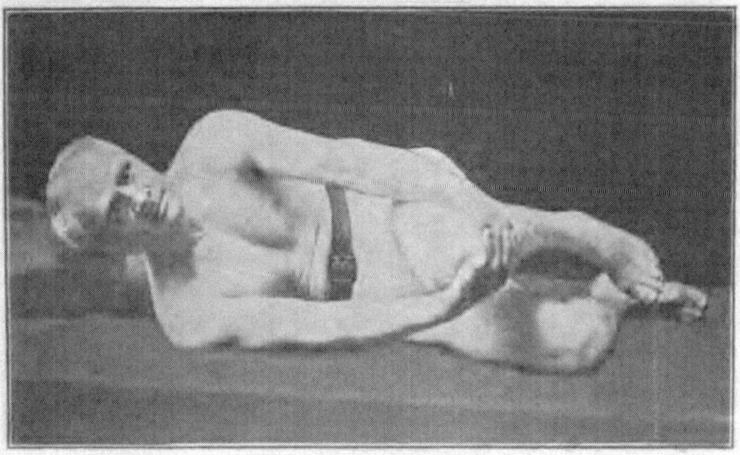

See Page 359. No. 22. Two Arm Pulling Exercise for Shoulders and Back. 5 Movements

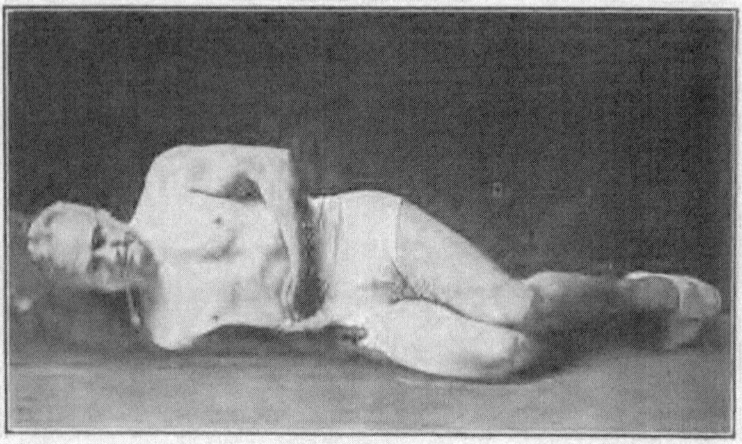

See Page 159. No. 23. Massage of Liver Lying Upon Right Side.
10 Movements

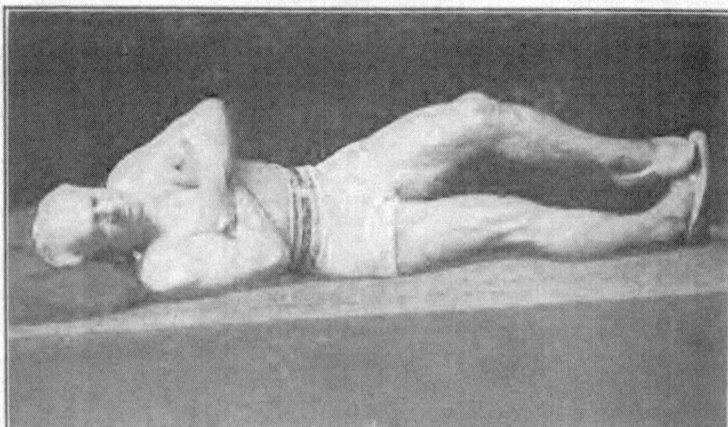

See Page 344. No. 24 Climbing Muscles of Legs 10 Movements, Alternately

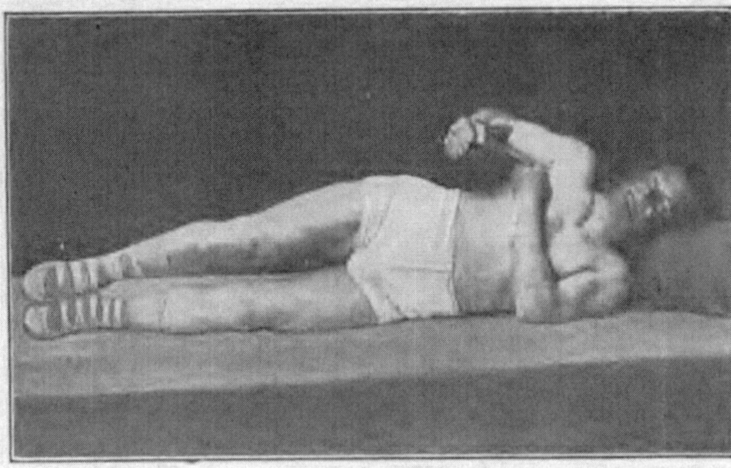

See Page 159. No. 25. Percussion of the Liver. 20 Light Blows

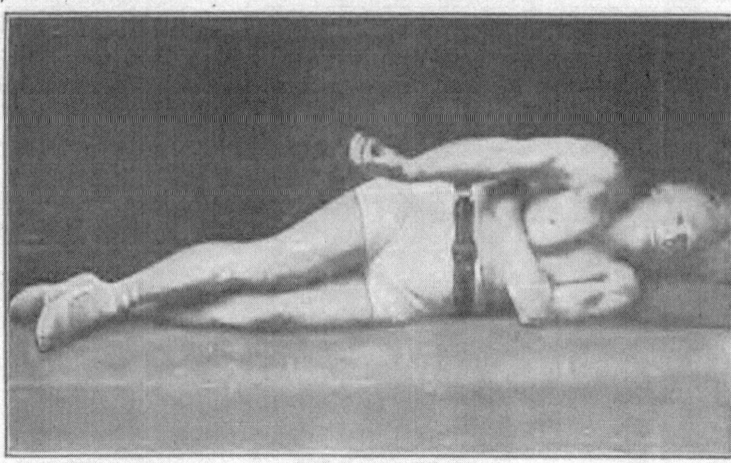

See Page 367. No. 26. Arm Twisting Exercise. 5 Movements

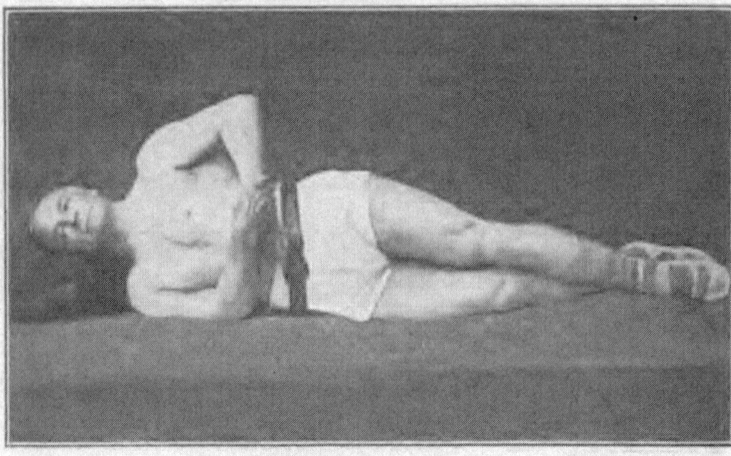

See Page 365. No. 27. Resistance Arm Exercise. 5 Movements

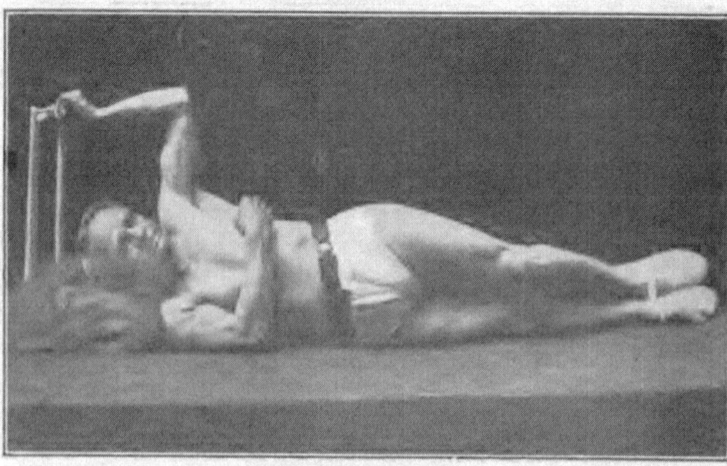

See Page 379. No. 28. Bar Exercise on Side, One Arm. 5 Movements

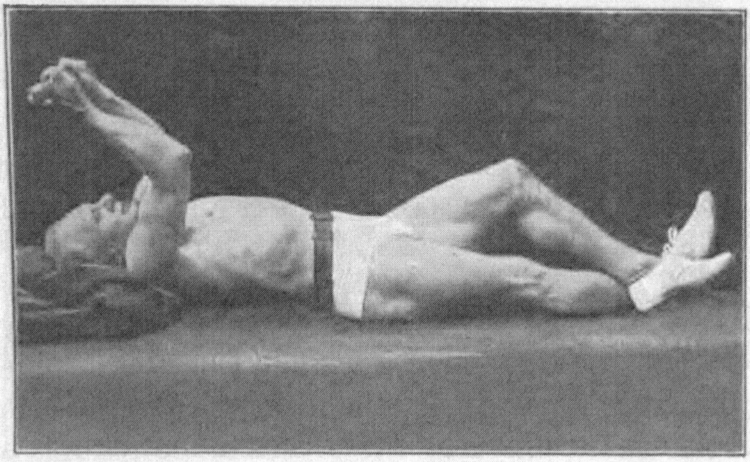

See Page 376. No. 29. Bar Exercise on Back, Two Arms. 5 Movements

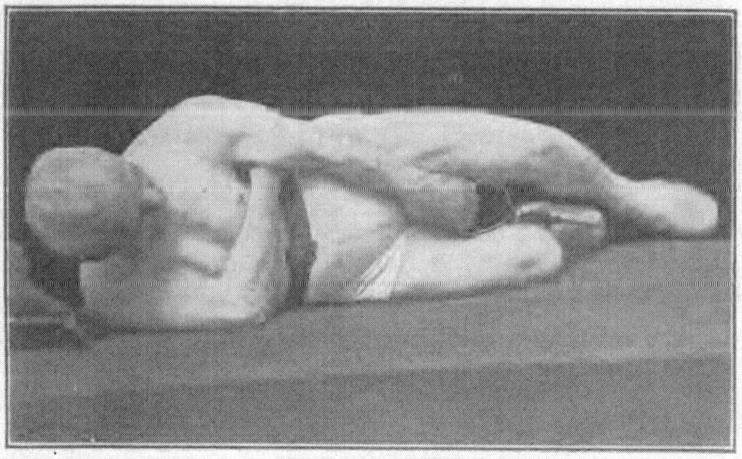

See Page 341. No. 30. Using the Lifting Board

Sunlight and Fresh Air

ALL energy surely emanates from the sun and without sunlight healthy conditions are impossible. There is no substitute, there can be none, for the sun is the only source of that all pervading force, the life principle, that mysterious form of energy which controls the universe, the governing power of this world. Therefore, if you would prolong your life stay in the sunlight as much as possible. If you wish to be healthy, breathe deeply fresh air charged with the sun's vitalizing rays. All forms of life are dependent upon solar energy, the sun being the great dynamo from which all life force is derived. It animates all vegetation and every form of life upon this earth. Sunshine really is life, without it, health is impossible and existence intolerable. Yet it must be admitted that vast numbers of people conduct their lives as though the human mechanism were an exception to that natural law. Pure air, which has been vitalized by sunshine, is charged with the vital principle, and it cannot be so vitalized by any other method, all pretentious assertions of alleged scientific discoveries in that direction are fallacious. Pure air is our greatest blessing and the foundation of health and longevity. The reader will probably say, "I know all this." Certainly you do, but the percentage of people who do not know it or who do not appreciate its value, you can easily find out by raising or attempting to raise a window in a crowded street car, and if you need an object lesson upon the value of sunlight, look at the pallid faces of the employees of our great sunless department stores or other indoor workers.

Regarding the benefits of deep breathing, *i. e.*, prolonged inhalations of pure air, it is true that the gross bulk of the air taken into the lungs does not penetrate through muscles, nerves and bones, but as it is charged with the vital principle or solar energy, the act of breathing sends everywhere through the body the electric fluid, the force which rebuilds and renews the mechanism of the system. Air which has been exposed to sunlight possesses the life principle to a far greater extent than the air of sunless rooms. In this connection and referring to the exercises I practice while lying in bed, I admit that it would be far better to go through them in the sunlight with its life-giving rays playing upon the naked body, but this is usually inconvenient and in my case especially so, therefore I practice this "lazy man's system of exercising" while lying in bed as the next best method, and my success in rejuvenating my old body at three score and ten, even with this disadvantage, is the best proof of the efficiency of my system. Many physical culture advocates and eager health seekers will approve the suggestion to exercise in a nude condition and in the sunshine, but urge the difficulty of putting it into practice.

To make this generally convenient and feasible within the next quarter of a century, I will present an architectural suggestion which, if once adopted, would surely be in vogue in all sanitariums or health resorts and also be adopted by municipalities with the view of improving the physical condition of dwellers in crowded cities. I hope the suggestion will be put in practice long before the end of that period. I suggest utilizing the roofs of all tenement or apartment houses by building thereon glass-enclosed rooms or solariums, just as the early Romans did, minus the glass. I further predict that this improvement will be generally adopted; that the health boards of progressive cities will see the value of such an arrangement and that something of this nature will be embodied in their building laws. If such a regulation were made a part of the building laws of any crowded city, it would be a great factor in improving the general health of its residents, and the mortality of that city would surely decrease. The poor of New York, dwellers in the crowded tenements of that great huddled-up beehive, have already recognized the value of the roofs of tenement buildings as health resorts and wherever possible throughout the heated term such roofs are used as dormitories at night and playgrounds by day; for though the small and usually badly-ventilated rooms of the building be hot and stuffy, a breeze is almost sure to be found on the roof. Even if there is none, the air there is purer than in the too often sunless rooms or in the crowded, narrow street below.

Through the efforts of Mr. Jacob Riis and his co-workers and many philanthropic organizations for the betterment of life in tenements, the proper sanitary conditions are compulsory and are usually well-regulated. But occupancy of the roofs as health resorts has not yet become general, although the improvement is evident and the necessity urgent. To those living in stuffy apartments or longing through the hot summer months for the presumably cooler breezes of the country, but unable to leave town, I will suggest a means by which this longing can be abated even in the most crowded sections and at small expense. Urge your landlords to utilize the roofs of apartment buildings as roof garden health resorts for their tenants. All health publications will endorse such a proposition and if the movement is once started it will soon become popular, for the benefits are too obvious to be overlooked. If the association of tenement workers will take the matter up methodically and persistently, newspapers and magazines generally will help, and when once the owners of this kind of property realize the folly of permitting this valuable space to lie idle and tenanted only by the sparrows, while buildings having such attractive improvements rent far more readily than those in which it is lacking, they will act and act promptly. To make the conditions ideal, such a house top health resort should be sheltered both top and sides, either wholly or in part, by glass. It must be as easy of access as the lower floors to make the innovation popular, and should be provided with conveniences for the care of the plants and flowers, which tenants would surely furnish and be glad of the opportunity to do so. The architectural details are simple, easily carried out, and in view of the great benefits and attraction of such an improvement, the cost would be comparatively small. Show your landlord this chapter and suggest that he bring the country into town, as far as his building is concerned. If he has been afflicted with many vacancies and is desirous of keeping his apartments always rented, he will realize that here is given the solution of the problem. Let him start such a roof garden and that building will never bear the familiar legend, "Rooms To Let," to which might well be added, "In hoc signo vinces."

Such an arrangement would be as attractive to the tenants of any building so improved, as are the parks and squares to the general public, and if properly and conveniently arranged, would to a very considerable extent satisfy the natural longing of all city dwellers for what are supposed to be the customary rural advantages: flowers, plants, pure air and sunshine, and this without many of the uncomfortable conditions often found in country life. There would be no necessity of abandoning home conveniences, your business need not be neglected, and you would have all this without the expense of your country vacation trips. Some day an architectural millenium will come to pass and the now vacant roof space will be converted into health resorts, breathing places for huddled-up city dwellers. After my own experiences in a lot of summer vacation failures in which the pleasant conditions described and which I expected to find existed largely in the imagination of the advertisers, I am convinced that they could have been more easily obtained and better at home by a roof garden of the kind in question. It is the old story of the cobbler in Aesop's fables, who journeyed far in search of wealth only to find it waiting for him at home in his own garden.

This is not a new idea, it is simply an adaptation of the methods of the early Romans with up-to-date conveniences. It was the usual architectural arrangement in those days and was then deservedly popular. Some day it will be equally in vogue here, but our climate is different, therefore the necessity of being glass sheltered and thus giving protection from winds and rain. Being a resident of San Francisco, I will add fogs. Life with such an arrangement could be made pleasant and healthful whatever the weather conditions might be outside. For anemic or consumptive people, for those advanced in years, indoor workers, or children, this is the ideal method for city dwellers. All life comes from the sun and such an architectural arrangement, if combined with rational exercise and cleanliness, both external and internal, and observance of the laws of hygiene, would be an important factor in the prolongation of life. The average city dweller of moderate circumstances need only recall some of his country vacations, and he will more readily appreciate the force of this suggestion. Most of you have experienced the discomforts often attending such a vacation. The annoyance of hot, crowded cars, the long and expensive trip, and when you arrived at your destination to find a woeful lack of conveniences resulted in a "wish-you-hadn't-come" feeling. To those who have suffered like me on such expeditions, I particularly address these remarks, and think that they will be appreciated. This roof-garden plan, if carried out properly, may to some extent reconcile you to stay in town, during summer vacation time anyhow. It would ensure some rural advantages which you might fail in finding, at least where "keeping summer boarders" is a means of livelihood.

But how about the views of the female members of the family? "It isn't fashionable." Well, not just now, but if this matter were systematically agitated, better architectural conditions would result and it soon would be a "fad," then, of course, fashionable. Laws regulating the construction of such structures may some day be enacted, but that architectural millennium will not arrive for some time, still it is safe to predict that before twenty years have elapsed, public opinion will agitate the enactment of a law requiring the construction of such health arrangements upon the roofs of all tenement buildings which will, I think, find favor with the officers of all health boards, as the benefits to the health of the tenants and the general health of the city would be obvious. The owners of the better class of buildings would soon install them, competition compelling them to do so. At present they all neglect the opportunity of utilizing this most valuable space of their buildings (the roofs), but this arrangement is so easy to construct and the advantages so great that it will not long be overlooked. It is remarkable that it has not become in vogue long ago.

If it is not considered desirable to utilize the entire space as a roof garden, convert a part of it into glass-covered rooms, both sides and roof, and the advantages of the "sunny front rooms" always featured in apartment advertisements will be "double discounted." Such rooms can be easily and effectively ventilated by transom devices, and if made as easy of access as the other lower apartments and provided with the same modern conveniences, will be very much more attractive than any other rooms in the building and will be eagerly sought after. The sunlight can be regulated by shades or screens, and as a renting proposition this would surely be profitable. To those unfortunates who are afflicted with the great "white plague," consumption, I confidently state, that in the sunny roof-garden can be found health conditions which will be a great factor towards their cure. If it is possible in your case to make such an arrangement, do so; it may save your life.

Quoting at length from an excellent pamphlet entitled "The Modern Crusade Against Consumption," by Prof. Irving Fisher, of New Haven, Conn., I submit the following valuable extracts and data: "No other disease, except pneumonia, has any death rate like it. The mortality from tuberculosis equals that from peritonitis, appendicitis, scarlet fever, typhoid fever, diphtheria, grippe, cancer and small-pox combined. In this country one person in nine dies of it and of the deaths which occur between the ages of 15 and 45, one-third are due to tuberculosis. In Germany, between the ages of 20 and 25, almost half of the deaths are from tuberculosis, a terrible exhibit, and this in the face of the hosts of alleged infallible medicinal remedies." The folly of it all! Neither medicines, diet, nor any form of hypodermic injections of alleged curative lymph discoveries, seem to be a "sure cure" for this terrible disease. They all have their season of advantage and possibly scientific publicity, then are forgotten and lapse into oblivion. Many cures are claimed for most of these discoveries, hence, the scientific endorsements, but when the evidence is carefully sifted down the curative process will usually be found to have resulted from a better method of living, improved sanitary conditions, out-of-door life, plenty of sunshine, fresh air, systematic exercise, cleanliness, and a rational system of diet. Given these conditions, with faith in the nostrum administered, for faith and courage are important factors, the chances of recovery are good, and this in spite of the abracadabra remedies and medicines taken. Again referring to Prof. Fisher's pamphlet, he says, "Naegli concludes an extended investigation with the statement that practically every adult has latent tuberculosis."

This means that each of us has a certain

number of bacilli encysted in the lungs waiting the opportunity to develop into this dread disease. With the resisting force of good health they are kept under control, but given the conditions of a lack of all the health factors enumerated and consequently lowered vitality, tuberculosis is not alone possible but probable. Consumption is now known to be a preventable disease; that is, where rational hygienic methods of life are followed and it can be cured by the modern out-of-door system now practiced in Colorado, Massachusetts and several other states; it is also in great favor in Germany and other parts of Europe. Not only is it a common disease, but it is an infectious disease, and this is another reason why the general public should be actively interested in its prevention and cure. It was formerly thought that consumption was the type of a hereditary disease and only specified classes of persons could have it. As a matter of fact, any kind of physique may be attacked when digestion and assimilation are defective, muscular inactivity usual and the most dangerous condition of all, a lack of sunshine and pure air. Under these conditions the peril of "the great white plague" is near. Reverse this order of things, live as I suggest, acquire resisting power, and you need not fear it, for a healthy body is a germ-killer apparatus. The disease is easily preventable and it is only because of the general ignorance and indifference that it has become so prevalent. Consumptives should have paper spit-cups, and with the expectorations should be burned daily. Spitting upon the floor should be prohibited, and the spitting ordinance strictly enforced, this especially applying to the corridors of post-offices, railway waiting-rooms or other much frequented public buildings. Out-of-doors and in the sunshine I do not believe infection to be so liable. It seems to be a parasitic disease and parasites do not thrive in sunlight. It spreads like a fire and like a fire can be easily extinguished in its incipiency, but when once beyond a certain point it cannot be extinguished. If there is any suspicion that the disease has been contracted, at once have a microscopic examination made of the expectorations; that is the only certain method of determining the presence of tubercular bacilli. If they are present, then act as I suggest and act promptly; there is no time to waste. The agency of cure was once thought to lie solely in good climate, but the many undeniable out-of-door cures to the credit of the various consumptive sanitariums which practice this excellent method in all kinds of weather, would seem to contradict that theory.

Again quoting from Prof. Fisher's pamphlet, "The patients sleep out-of-doors even in winter." Of course during that season they are sheltered overhead, but whether it snows, rains or freezes, in a very short time they usually seem to enjoy "sleeping out," and for the most part soon present a very improved condition. I am confident that this method of cure is possible in almost any climate and it is certainly rapidly gaining in vogue, but until the old prejudices against night air and drafts are overcome, it will not become general. Another obstacle is, that while it is an excellent remedy for consumptives, it is rather a drawback upon the science of making a living by giving medicines for its cure, hence it is gaining favor slowly. The treatment does not consist in fresh air alone, but of four principal factors, viz.: air cure, food cure, rest cure and mind (or faith) cure. The only criticism I make is, that they do not seem to rely so much upon sunshine as the other advantages enumerated. I predict, however, that ultimately it will be found that sunshine is the greatest factor of all in the curative process, the sine qua non. I do not undervalue in any way the wonderful invigorating powers of the climate of Colorado, as I have tried it long ago and know its value, but I have more faith in the virtues of sunshine and fresh air. These you can always find upon the roof of any city building and if the glass rooms I have suggested are constructed, you will have a sanitarium at home in which, with side screens, you may effectively practice the exercises I describe in a nude condition, and this under the most favorable of all health conditions, in the sunshine. Practice them systematically and persistently and success will be yours. For the rest, eat such nourishing food as agrees with you. There is no set rule to a diet, as every stomach seems to have different requirements. Chew thoroughly each mouthful, as Horace Fletcher suggests; Bathe frequently, Keep the colon (the lower bowel) clean (see chapter upon internal cleanliness), Determine that you will get well and you will, if you follow my advice and stick to it. Hunt up some pleasant-mannered Christian Scientist practitioner and add his or her assurances of your recovery. As I have before stated, I am not a Christian Scientist, at least from a religious standpoint, but I have great faith in it or any other harmless method which will inspire confidence, courage and hope, for these are the great factors of cure in all diseases. Your trusted family physician may do, if he will confine his medical prescriptions to bread pills or other harmless medical abracadabra, but to succeed, he must inspire confidence and carry out the simple but effective system I outline. Unfortunately, if trained in old school doctrines, he will be so thoroughly saturated with those antiquated teachings that, like the chef who resigned from a highly-paid job rather than to cook without garlic, the worthy M.D. will probably abandon the case, declining to adopt the methods of a layman whose teachings, according to his ideas, savor of heresy. But I know what I am talking about. My father died of consumption at 42. I inherited his physical disabilities and throughout my sickly, feeble babyhood, boyhood and early manhood, everyone interested in me predicted that I would certainly go as my father did. And so I would had I followed the same antiquated fool methods and alleged medicinal remedies then practiced, and are to a great extent still in vogue with the medical profession. The unprecedented instance of my physical improvement and rejuvenation at 72, after the unfavorable conditions under which my life commenced, is the best proof of the sanity of my methods and the benefits resultant therefrom. There is, however, one point upon which I heartily agree with the orthodox medical profession, and this is, that in a case of severe sickness you should at once engage a trained nurse, one knowing the laws of hygiene, understanding the use of sick-room conveniences, and versed in the gentle, helpful methods of modern, scientific nursing. If in your emergency you can find such a one who has the courage to practice her profession without the shadow of a drug store doctor's presence to interfere with her helpful ministrations, engage her at once, then hoist your flag and read your declaration of independence to the entire medical profession, which includes the sympathetic commission drug stores. As a starter in the new order of things pull up the blinds of your sunless family vaults, the "guest chamber" and. the equally depressing front parlor. This will give the sunshine a chance to destroy any germs of consumption which may be keeping house there. "But the flies will come in and the new carpet will be faded." Sure they will, but a new carpet will cost less than the doctor's bill and it is just possible you would rather have a sun-faded carpet than to have your neighbors gather in that sunless parlor or depressing guest chamber and say, "Poor dear, how natural he looks, and he had the best doctor and the best medicine that money could procure." That is the way my father went. Don't go that way, try Nature's method. I have tried to make it clear and hope you will appreciate its value.

The Fasting Cure

AS I have previously stated, the matter I present in this book generally relates to my own experiences in the science of physical rejuvenation, giving in detail the simple means by which I have accomplished that fortunate condition, but this chapter principally concerns the experiences of others who have more extensively experimented in the method of curing bodily ailments by "The Fasting Cure." The great success which has resulted in several cases practiced under my immediate observation, as well also of many cases whose authenticity I have every reason to believe, has caused me to investigate the matter to the best of my ability. To this authenticated data, I have added my own personal, if limited, experiences of the benefits resulting from fasting for a few days only.

Forty years ago I sang a great deal in public, a part of my income being derived from the concerts in which I appeared and the church choirs in which I was engaged. A bad cold, therefore, was not alone a physical inconvenience, but a financial loss, as in that condition I was unable to keep my musical engagements, or if I did, appeared at a great disadvantage. In those days I implicitly believed in the curative powers of medicines and had great faith in the old adage of "stuff a cold and starve a fever." Therefore, when I "caught cold" it always meant a long period of inaction as a singer, for I recovered very slowly from such attacks.

I had been engaged to sing at a fashionable concert in which I very much wanted to appear. The papers were full of the affair, the programs were printed, and the theater had been long engaged. Then three days before the event that "bete noir" of all singers made its appearance. I "caught an awful cold." It is not necessary to recite the symptoms. You all know them. I had not much "resisting power" at that age, and from my past experiences I knew that that cold would inevitably grow worse and I should be unable to sing. In my distress, I called upon the manager of the affair and stated my dilemma. He was an eminent surgeon in those days, but had even then as little faith in the curative powers of medicines as I have now. As I was raised upon the old "stuff-a-cold-and-starve-a-fever" doctrine, I very naturally mentioned it as my intended remedy, admitting, however, that I was apparently "in for a siege." He wagged his blessed old gray head and said: "I know you want to sing, young man, and sing you can; that is, if you will accept my remedy for a cold. I always successfully try it when I am afflicted as you are, and I always speedily recover. It is not popular now, but some day it will be. Starve! Starve! Starve! Drink all the water you can, but do not take food of any description. Continue this treatment until that 110 pulse of yours goes down to 72 and your 103 temperature gets back to 98. I think this will happen before the end of three days, possibly sooner, and when it does, I shall expect you to show up at the theater and sing as you are billed. Now you go home and soak yourself in as hot a bath as you can stand, put a couple of mild porous plasters upon your chest and two between your shoulders. Go to bed and stay there until I tell you to get up, and don't take any medicines. Your family doctor and anxious relatives will certainly insist that you must take some nourishment. They will probably think you are insane if you refuse—"your strength must be kept up, as death might result from weakness," etc., etc. But it will not do anything of the kind. Don't be afraid. You do as I tell you, then you will appear as you have agreed to do. 'Stuff a cold and starve a fever' be hanged. You have a fever now—a pretty bad one, and it is going to be worse; that is, if you do not follow my advice. All you need is sufficient courage and determination to follow it and follow it to the letter. You will not grow weak for lack of nourishment in a three days' fast, and you couldn't digest food anyhow with such a fever. You are billed to sing and you must appear."

I took his advice. The results were exactly as he had stated. At the end of the three days' fast I made a satisfactory afternoon rehearsal, and successfully sang my numbers the same night, and this without a trace of the bad cold! As my past experiences had led me to expect a month's siege, the fasting cure was a revelation!

Now that is my experience of fasting for even a few days, and that is how I have cured my bad colds ever since for the past forty years. I have given the same advice to many singers, but like "angels' visits" those who have followed it are "few and far between."

The demonstrated truth is, that fasting does cure colds and it cures them quickly, and you don't have to "take something for it." It isn't a popular remedy, at least not just now, but it is Nature's effective cure for glandular troubles, such as colds are, and I think the only effective method of curing a cold.

If I were a practicing physician I would urgently advise it, even if I had the entire local medical fraternity "down on me" for doing so. It is "unprofessional advice" and too cheap and easy anyway, and I would probably suffer a loss of patients; *i. e.*, if I had any.

But then, you see, I don't practice and have only one patient—myself. I have made quite a success of him and that is all that I ever intended to do. It is too much trouble to give verbal advice and more to answer letters; that is why I write this book. You will find all my health methods in it, and the next time you catch a cold try the remedy I have described. It is perfectly safe, not unpleasant and you will save money in medicines, doctors' bills and, incidentally, meals.

My old friend has "passed over" long since, but he has my hearty thanks for the good advice he gave me forty years ago, and I sincerely hope that residential conditions with him are of a nature which will enable him to hear of my gratitude. My opinion is, that if he were alive, he would surely be the author of a book upon fasting as valuable as any of these I will presently name and recommend. If you are interested in these books they will give you more explicit details than I can present in my limited space. The advice and data that you will then find are very valuable. Anyhow, fasting is the method I practice to cure a bad cold and one of the reasons why my singing voice, a very high and powerful concert baritone, is as good at seventy-two as it was at thirty-two.

We all eat too much; that is, unless restricted by financial stringency, and excess in eating may be said to be almost universal. That custom, combined with hurried eating and lack of sufficient mastication, is the cause of say eighty per cent. of digestive disorders. I leave out the other twenty per cent. to be charged up to tobacco, "treats" and "I'm in a hurry to get back to the office." But all this does not seem to apply to boys. I have arrived at that conclusion after trying to fill up several hungry small boys. I don't know where they stowed that dinner or what they did with it, but they couldn't be filled. Therefore, I except hungry boys.

I have received many letters asking about my system of diet. Now, I am going to make a confession. I haven't any. I eat whatever I like, and lots of it. My excuse is that I have a ravenous small-boy appetite and am proud of it. That appetite is due to continuous systematic exercise, resulting in activity of all organs, both digestive and glandular, and any food that I take is eaten slowly and thoroughly chewed. Under these conditions the process of assimilation and elimination are upon a healthy equilibrium, therefore the perfect health I enjoy at over "three score and ten."

Incidentally, I will remark that this satisfactory digestive condition cannot be acquired by any dinner pills or other digestive stimulants, all advertisements to the contrary. You may temporarily stimulate the digestive process by such methods, but sooner or later there will be a reaction. Nature will object and finally when your stomach goes on a protracted strike you will "wish you hadn't." And when in the hurry and struggle for financial success that most important of all organs of the human mechanism breaks down, life will not be worth living. "For what if a man gain the whole world and lose"—his stomach?

For myself I couldn't have a better appetite or digestion. But if I were lacking in that respect I would fast occasionally for a few days just to give my stomach a rest and if I had a fever, catarrhal trouble or a "bad cold," or any other glandular disorder (for that is what a bad cold is) I would rely upon the fasting method to cure them. I will go farther than this: I believe that both pneumonia and appendicitis in their first stages can be almost certainly cured by a longer treatment, adopting the same system as that described in my three days' fasting experience, adding to that treatment, however, thorough flushing of the colon (or large bowel; see details of this method in chapter headed "Internal Cleanliness"). Also add the gentle ministrations of a thoroughly-trained professional nurse, and the absent treatment of any drug-store doctor. Under these conditions a satisfactory cure is almost certain. In neglected cases of appendicitis, of course, the knife of an able surgeon is the only remedy, but only in extreme cases. Usually the patient in an appendicitis operation should be labeled "Opened by Mistake," and then be pasted together again. After this has been done the conditions are similar to Messrs. Peary's and Cook's claims of discovery of the North Pole—the correctness of the diagnosis can neither be proven nor disproven.

The results of my investigations of methods by which Nature cures is that short fasts at intervals are important factors in preserving health and therefore of prolonging life. And I firmly believe that in nearly all forms of disease "fasting" is a most effective remedy. Really the short fasts which are a part of the Catholic and Jewish religions must have had their origin in the discovery of the beneficial effects of totally abstaining from all food at stated periods. I am a Jew and a Catholic to that extent. As to the logical reasons for sometimes resting the digestive organs, if the most confirmed dyspeptic had driven a horse until it was exhausted he would know enough to stop and give it a rest. But it never seems to occur to that dyspeptic cripple that the same rule applies to his own stomach. Instead of resting it he seeks relief in alleged dyspepsia remedies or alcoholic stimulants. These only temporarily relieve his distress. Reaction follows and he is usually worse off than he was before. As a reformed dyspeptic with over thirty years of personal experience in alleged medicinal remedies for that infernal complaint, I have seen the error of my ways. My recovery is principally due to practicing the same simple means by which you permitted your tired horse to regain his strength; that is, I have at intervals given my exhausted digestive organs short rests. In other words, when my familiar old malady reappeared I have fasted for two or three days, and always with good results. It is Nature's simple, inexpensive, but most effective remedy. Any four-footed fool jackass knows enough to practice that remedy when his stomach is on a strike. But his two-footed fool dyspeptic master doesn't.

My advice, if your stomach is out of order, is to do what the jackass does—fast for two or three days. If your case of dyspepsia is bad and chronic, two or three days more will make a better job of it. But don't do too much at once. I think several short fasts are better than one long one. As an instance of the ease and small inconvenience attendant upon a long fast and the benefits derived from it, I present the case of Mr. John A. Wilson, a prominent member of the Berkeley (California) City Council. This gentleman had been long afflicted with a serious case of nasal catarrh, other complications being imminent. All orthodox remedies had been unavailingly tried, the sufferer had almost given up hope of being cured, and tried the fasting cure as a last resort. After thoroughly studying the method he carefully prepared himself for a 30 days' trial. This he commenced upon the evening of the 1st day of October, 1911. It ended successfully in public before an audience of about one thousand persons at the Berkeley Auditorium, Tuesday evening, October 31st, 1911. Owing to the political prominence of this gentleman, the Press of San Francisco, as well as of Berkeley and many other cities, have given this fast a great deal of publicity; also considerable controversy has arisen between members of the medical profession who oppose fasting and those advocating its benefits.

Under these conditions my statement of the case may be of interest to the reader. I was engaged to deliver a lecture upon my methods of physical rejuvenation at the Berkeley Auditorium the same date; *i. e.*, October 31st, 1911. I appeared upon the stage with Mr. Wilson and had every opportunity to acquaint myself with his physical condition at the end of this thirty days' fast. Throughout that period I also met him frequently and examined his pulse, temperature and general condition. Quite a number of the medical profession and press representatives also availed themselves of the same privilege. There was no question of the honesty and strict observance of an absolute fast for the period of thirty days, and it is only after Mr. Wilson has satisfactorily demonstrated the benefits of the experiment that any adverse criticism has been publicly made, and this only by interested opponents of Nature's remedy.

It has been publicly stated that Mr. Wilson's health has been impaired by the long abstinence from food. Answering this, I have met him frequently since his fast and he assures me that he is healthier than he has been for twenty years, and he looks it. The chronic catarrh has wholly disappeared, and my opinion is that he is now a very healthy man. It has been stated that he was very weak when he appeared upon the stage upon the evening of October 31st. If he was, then, to use an Irishism, he must have been "powerful weak," as he insisted upon carrying my valise, full of books and other heavy matter, weighing in all forty-nine pounds, for the space of two blocks. And this four hours before he appeared with me upon the stage. His eye was clear, pulse regular and strong, and he walked beside me with the same steady rapidity which is my customary gait. If you wish to know the significance of that strength test try to carry forty-nine pounds two blocks without resting. It was a revelation to me.

In answer to a letter of inquiry as to his physical condition, he replied, under date of December 2nd, 1911: "My weight before my 30 days' fast was 165 pounds and now is 160. I lost during the October fast 19 pounds and regained 14 pounds in November. My age is sixty years; my height, 5 feet 9½ inches. I am in perfect health—better than before, but I think the most important thing I learned was confidence in my ability to take care of myself and of preserving my health by this method."

My summary of the matter is that the difference between systematic fasting, *i. e.*, voluntary abstinence from all food with a definite curative object in view, and enforced involuntary fasting (that is starvation) lies wholly in the mental attitude. I make this statement as I have tried both methods and speak from experience. During the latter part of 1868 and a few months in 1869 I was engaged by the *Chicago Tribune* and some other parties financially interested in the construction of The Kansas Pacific R. R. to go to the end of the line and report periodically all matters relating to the enterprise. This hastily-constructed, flimsy affair was stranded near Fort Wallace, somewhere near the center of Kansas. The country was a vast treeless rolling prairie, tenanted by predatory Cheyenne Indians, buffalo, antelope, prairie dogs and rattlesnakes. Just the country in which a greenhorn was likely to lose himself and unlikely to be found again alive. I went along with one of the surveying parties and was no exception to the greenhorn custom. I stalked a small herd of buffalo near camp, and in the course of an hour suddenly realized that either the sun was in the wrong place or I was hopelessly lost. The awful sense of despair attendant upon this discovery almost paralyzed me. I couldn't reason out the way back and remembering the fate of other lost greenhorns had but little hope, as there were no trees or landmarks to guide me. I had quietly left camp before day-break, and as the surveyors came in only at night there would be no possible chance for a rescue until the next day. I wandered on until I fell from exhaustion. That day passed into the next and the next, and then at the end of the fourth day I was found by our scouts, delirious, staggering blindly along and wasted to a bag of bones. It took me a month to recover from that experience, and yet I have frequently voluntarily fasted two or three days and several times as long as four days, without loss of strength, with little loss of flesh and no after effects other than of benefit.

My summary of the matter is, as I have stated, that the difference between starving and fasting lies in the mental attitude and the beneficial effect of fasting is that it gives the stomach needed rest in any digestive disorders, while in "bad colds" the clogging rubbish or surplus matter is burned up or eliminated from the body and glandular structures very much in the same way that end is accomplished by prolonged systematic exercise.

The result in all of my experiences has been wonderfully beneficial. I have made but little preparation for my short fasts. I simply stopped eating and followed the plan hereinbefore described. At the end of these three or four days I always ate a light meal of well-cooked vegetables and the next day almost created a household famine by my vigorous appetite. Space will not permit me to describe the details and preparation for an extended fast such as Mr. Wilson made, and I prefer to refer you to the books written by able specialists upon this important matter. If I did write those details I would be accused of copying them. The information you require will be found in "The True Science of Living," by Edward Hooker Dewey, M.D., published by Charles C. Haskell & Co., Norwich, Conn., and "The Fasting Cure," by Upton Sinclair, sold by Physical Culture Publishing Co., New York. Price, $1.00.

The only danger in the fasting system, if not of too long duration, seems to lie at its termination. Taper off gently and don't gorge yourself. Do this and no harm will result. At the end of my four days' fasts I have taken, in moderation, grape juice, well boiled rice and green peas and carrots, the next day anything I liked, provided I chewed it.

Regarding my strictures upon the drug store medical profession: I am but voicing the opinion of a great rising tide of intelligent protest against such antiquated methods. Alleged medicinal remedies, long in favor, are losing their popularity. The halo of the old style, drug-dosing allopathic physician is out of fashion and dingy. Patent medicines require more advertising than formerly—dupes are not so plentiful and the pure food law has had a very discouraging effect upon that industry. In short, people are commencing to think, to learn more of Nature's effective methods of cure and appreciate their value. As a .result, the familiar sign, "Drugs" will be unfashionable before the end of this century. The advance is slow but it is sure. As far as you are concerned, as a means of health, learn all you can of Nature's effective cure for digestive disorders, colds and most minor glandular troubles. My space will not admit of all of the details you will require, but the authors of the books named are authorities in the matter and I advise you to get those books. The "Physical Culture Magazine" of New York gives a great deal of space to the system and you will find much valuable data there. It is the pioneer publication in popularizing Nature's curative methods, and should be added to your sources of information upon a matter which should be of vital interest to you, *i. e.*, "The Fasting Cure."

The Secret of Good Digestion

DIGESTION of food begins in the mouth, and to accomplish perfectly this part of digestion the food must be thoroughly chewed, and in that process thoroughly insalivated. This will depend upon the condition of the tools you work with. Food cannot be thoroughly chewed unless the teeth are in good condition, and every tooth lost or diseased diminishes the ability of that person to masticate his food to the extent of that lost chewing surface. You might as well expect a carpenter to turn out a good job with few and poor tools as to expect your stomach to satisfactorily digest a lot of food which by reason of poor teeth, or few of them, was not sufficiently chewed. The loss of a tooth is therefore a misfortune, as just to that extent the preparatory process of digestion is crippled. If digestion is not perfect, and if assimilation is not perfect, health is impossible.

More bodily ills are due to what we eat and how we eat it, than any other cause. All the long train of digestive disorders, in fact, the majority of most human diseases, may be traced to the same basic starting point: What

9

you eat, how much you eat, and how you eat it, but principally the latter.

It is in the mouth that the first and one of the most important steps in digestion takes place; the only step, in fact, over which the individual has the slightest control, hence the importance in nutrition of sound teeth, a full supply, and a clean mouth. To believe as many do, that artificial teeth are quite as satisfactory in the mastication of food as natural ones, is a mistake. They sustain the same relation to natural teeth that a wooden leg does to one of flesh and bones, but if you lose a tooth, at once make good the loss by replacing it with an artificial one.

In this era of ingenious dentistry and really artistic bridgework, the counterfeit will do excellent service and will readily pass inspection. That is, unless you ask the interested investigator to "step inside." If you do not commit that indiscretion and the investigator is not a dentist, nobody will find out. However, it is just as well to remember the old Spanish proverb, "The man with a paste diamond shuns the society of Lapidaries," and apply it to your own case. But if through any great loss of your teeth a plate has been found necessary, do not hesitate to put it in and do so at once. For remember, "the stomach has no teeth," and if you have no teeth you will be unable to chew your food, therefore indigestion with all its miseries will surely result. Economize in any other direction you please but do not economize at a point where the process of nutrition commences. That would be "Penny wise and pound foolish." If a tooth is found to be decaying have it filled at once, as decay in its beginning can be easily arrested, without in the least impairing the usefulness of the tooth and early treatment is also less painful and less expensive. Usually the latter is a prime argument in its favor. Most people will not consult a dentist until they are really in pain. To avoid trouble have your teeth inspected at intervals, just as it is the custom to inspect elevators and boilers. It is less expensive in the "long run." What would be thought of the owner of a building who never had his elevators inspected, say at least two or three times a year?

Always keep the teeth clean. The time at which it is most necessary to cleanse the mouth and teeth is at bedtime. Really the ideal way to do this is after each meal. That is what I do, first using dental floss silk and this I always carry in my pocket. For convenience it is always put up in small, flat tin discs, manufactured and sold under the name "Red Cross Packet Dental Floss Silk." All druggists have them in stock, or should have. Draw the thread between the teeth, afterwards brush well.

Mornings and evenings I use a tooth paste put up in the ordinary sheet lead tubes, but instead of the usual round orifice or vent, get the kind with the narrow oblong vent. The paste comes out like a ribbon, it lasts longer, does not waste, and is far more cleanly. Don't keep any decayed teeth in your mouth; they are dangerous. Fill, crown, or if too badly decayed, and as a last resort, have them extracted; but don't let any teeth stay in your mouth that are decayed; they are dangerous. Decaying teeth spell Dyspepsia.

"Proper care of the mouth and teeth is one of the most important of all the measures that are taken for the protection of the human body and a failure to give them proper care is, in my judgment, the direct cause of more disease in the human family than any other single cause."

Major W. O. Owen, M.D., Surgeon U. S. Army, says, and to which I say Amen: "In tuberculosis, a great handicap is defective teeth, as such chewing tools make it impossible to properly masticate and assimilate food, therefore in all such cases see that the teeth are kept in good order. This is important as well as a well-nourished body is of the first importance in the prevention or cure of 'The Great White Plague,' and I am certain that a foul mouth and decaying teeth, especially in children, decidedly increases the chance of catching that dread disease as well as scarlet fever, diphtheria, measles or other contagious diseases. Under the most favorable conditions the human mouth may be regarded as an almost ideal culture medium for germ life. In fact, it presents in point of moisture, temperature, nutritive material, etc., an almost perfect breeding place for dangerous germs. As this condition exists under the most sanitary conditions, what must be expected when through neglect the teeth are decayed, the mouth foul, the breath offensive and the general situation a pertinacious invitation to dangerous bacilli."

Regarding the importance of mouth hygiene and care of the teeth, Dr. William Osler says: "There is not any one single thing more important in the whole range of hygiene, than the hygiene of the mouth. If I were asked to say whether more physical deterioration was produced by alcohol or by defective teeth, I should unhesitatingly say 'defective teeth'." He is all wrong in his chloroform statement, but surely all right in this.

In brief, dental diseases always mean, of whatever nature, an unclean and unhealthy mouth, but they mean more than that, and this is an important thing to be remembered. They are indirectly the basic cause of digestive disorders and often of the various contagious diseases.

You will admit that all of this is logical.

You can't help it. That is, if you consider the matter carefully. But then a great many people who read this stuff will say, "What a lot of bother." Of course it is; but this bother with a lot of my other methods of getting young again, are the reasons why at 72 I look not very much over half of my age. Which reminds me that upon one of my camping-out trips a dirty, sickly fellow we had with us said to me, as he watched me scrubbing away at my teeth, "You are a great trouble to yourself, ain't you?" Certainly, I admit it; that is why I am in such splendid health. And when any germs come loafing around my mouth, they decide not to apply for apartments, and instead they hunt up some such fellow, owning a lot of decayed teeth, a filthy mouth and a breath like a buzzard. Then they promptly move in and get busy. Later on that kind of a fellow is usually under a doctor's care and has to "take something for it." What he needed was a dentist and a tooth brush, then it would not have happened.

And now to fathers and mothers. If all this is too much trouble for yourselves, how about your children? Their young lives are dependent on you. They cannot help themselves and you are the responsible parties. All that I have said applies to those children and to a greater degree than to grown people. Remember that foul mouth and decaying teeth, particularly in children, decidedly increase the chances of catching contagious and infectious diseases, such as scarlet fever, diphtheria, measles and tuberculosis, and just remember that a clean mouth will do much to prevent such contagion.

"As a result of bad teeth and unsanitary mouths the physical development of a growing child is seriously retarded. The more the physical development is disturbed the less in general is the mental capacity. Therefore the more defective the teeth, also the worse, as a rule, is the school standing." I quote this from an excellent work upon "School Hygiene and Discipline."

As a summary, sound teeth properly used are an absolute necessity to good digestion, and in your efforts to cure your dyspepsia the first thing you should do should be to put your chewing tools in order, and having done so, keep them in that condition. At your meals use them thoroughly and deliberately, don't hurry, for if you do you will not make a good job of it and if you don't make a good job of this preparatory process and bolt your food, you will regret it. Food must be thoroughly chewed or properly assimilated before it is taken into the stomach, and as "the stomach has no teeth," it cannot be chewed there. As a consequence it will remain too long in the digestive tract, there it will rot and dyspepsia, acid stomach, flatulency and the train of evils which follow indigestion will result. Medicines do not cure that condition; they may temporarily allay the distress, but if you bolt your food you may expect the trouble back again at your next meal, medicine or no medicines. I suffered from the agonies of acute dyspepsia for thirty years, and only recovered after I had learned to eat slowly and chew my food thoroughly. That is the secret of my present excellent digestion.

Don't bother with pre-digested foods or alleged dyspepsia cures. Take my advice, first as to putting your chewing tools in order, and how to keep them in that condition, then learn how to eat.

To the best of my belief Horace Fletcher did not invent the art of chewing food, but he performed a great service to mankind when he iterated and reiterated his advice to chew food thoroughly before it is placed in the stomach. He has written so exhaustively upon the subject that about all I can add to his advice is to get your chewing tools in order and at your meals use them thoroughly, and eat slowly; that is the great secret of a good stomach. If you have dyspepsia go without solid foods at your breakfast. Digestion is very slow when you are sleeping and there may be some residue from your last evening's meal; if there is that will hinder digestion of the next meal. If you are accustomed to drink coffee, weak tea or milk at your breakfast, and they agree with you, continue the practice, but not even a crust of bread. Any solid food will start the grinding process of the stomach muscles, for that is the next stage after food has been swallowed.

In the following chapter upon dyspepsia you will find described my methods of strengthening the stomach muscles, and it is important.

Dyspepsia

MOST people are afflicted with some form of digestive disorder, the "quick lunch habit" of the modern business man being more largely responsible for this condition than anything else; for it is not so much what you eat, as how you eat it. If your food is not thoroughly chewed, and, in that process, thoroughly insalivated, it will certainly be digested with difficulty when it reaches the stomach; and if this habit of swallowing the food hastily, and without proper mastication, is persisted in dyspepsia, with its various complications, will surely result.

There is no exception. Nature is a stern creditor, resenting any infraction of her laws. If you violate them, you will certainly suffer for it. And the severest penalties she inflicts are for transgressing the laws of digestion. Under the familiar title, dyspepsia, we group various distressing digestive disorders, most of which could be avoided by properly chewing the food.

I have stated that, in my personal experience, and by the system of exercises I practice, I have found it to be possibie to build up the aged human body after it has passed the half-century limit, and to restore to it the muscular development it may have possessed in earlier years; and that it is also possible to excel that condition. But this cannot be done when serious digestive disorders exist; until they are remedied improvement will be slow. As the trouble is usually caused by hurried eating and, consequently, insufficient mastication, the logical remedy is to take more time at meals, and chew the food thoroughly. This change in habits alone will, most probably, greatly improve the digestive conditions in a short time.

The next step is to strengthen the muscles of the stomach, for the digestion of food depends largely upon the strength of those muscles.

In the process of digestion, the muscles of the stomach alternately contract and relax, producing a churning motion which, with the aid of the digestive fluids, digests the food. Now, if those muscles are weak, the work of digestion will be carried on poorly and with great effort. If this process of digestion were solely the result of chemical action, then a healthy condition might, possibly, be artificially brought about by medicinal preparations, and cures might be effected by some of the numerous dyspepsia "dopes" advertised throughout the world. But, as muscular strength cannot be obtained from any drug, it is certain that these preparations cannot be the infallible remedies for digestive disorders the inventors and their advertisements claim for them. Temporary relief from the distress of indigestion may undoubtedly be obtained from these alleged remedies, and a more careful attention to diet—which the sufferer would most probably observe when taking them—would result in some improvement; but as well expect a cure by the use of opium, or any other anodyne, as to place dependence solely upon any drug, or combination of drugs.

The remedy lies with one's self, and, if the following brief directions are followed faithfully and persistently, any one will succeed as I have done.

Chew your food slowly, that it may be thoroughly insalivated and digested readily. It is also necessary to strengthen the muscles of the stomach. This can be accomplished by the following simple and easily-performed exercise:

Lying on your back, bend your head well forward. (This action will contract and tense the abdominal muscles.) When the head is dropped back to the horizontal position, those muscles will relax.

These alternate contraction and relaxation exercises will, of themselves, materially strengthen the muscles; but percussion will greatly aid in producing that result. Therefore, as you alternately raise and lower the head, and thus contract and relax the muscles, strike the abdomen rapidly with your clenched fists, at first lightly, but afterwards increasing the force of the blow, as the muscles become stronger. This exercise will direct the blood to that part, will produce a healthy circulation, and strengthen the digestive organs.

Another excellent exercise is to place the palms of the hands firmly upon the abdomen and rub back and forth, much in the way a washboard is used. These two exercises will also reduce any fatty deposit which may have accumulated, and are harmless, inexpensive, and far more effective than the most widely-advertised and most lauded "dyspepsia cures."

I speak from experience, as I suffered from dyspepsia for over thirty years, vainly seeking relief during all that time, from the various medicinal remedies prescribed by physicians, or others which I was induced to purchase by advertisements or by the recommendation of sympathetic friends.

The causes of my trouble were hurried meals, insufficient mastication, and weakness of the abdominal muscles. My cure was effected by the system I have described. To those unfortunates who are afflicted as I have been, I strongly urge the practice of these exercises for strengthening the abdominal muscles.

How I Strengthened My Eyes

THE loss of all of our faculties is equivalent to death, and the loss of any one of them brings you that much nearer the end. The loss of your hearing or your powers of locomotion is a great misfortune, but the greatest physical calamity which can befall one is the total loss of sight. All the wealth in the world will not offset such a misfortune. And I have been so near that condition that even the memory of those days still gives me the blues, the year "when the light failed." Always fearing a possible return to that awful condition, I am now as careful of my eyes as I was formerly negligent. Naturally, I had unusually good, strong eyes and that, I think, was the only point in my physical heritage in which I was not a weakling.

As I have elsewhere stated, in my younger days I was an accountant, an indoor sedentary profession which undermined my health and finally seriously injured my eyes. The consequence was that for a long time I knew the misery of being unable to read, unable to bear the sunlight, and as any ray of light was agony I stumbled about wearing very dark glasses, so dark that all the world seemed to be in a dim, uncertain twilight.

By a long enforced rest I partially recovered, but at about the time of my physical breakdown or when I had reached the age of fifty the trouble again commenced, but I was commencing to learn something, and that something was that any muscle or set of muscles, if exercised, will increase in size, strength and elasticity. Therefore, I reasoned, if this applied to the muscles of the body generally why would it not apply to the muscular structure of the eyes? I found that the action of each eye was controlled by six muscles, these being attached to the eye-balls and from them extended and attached to the bony structure in which they are encased. In the event of the reader wishing to read up on this subject you will find these muscles described about as follows:

The Superior Rectus, which moves the eye upward; the Inferior Rectus, which moves the eye downward; the Interior Rectus, which moves the eye inward; the Exterior Rectus, which moves the eye outward; the Superior and Inferior Oblique muscles, which control the rotation of the eye-ball. This is copied from an elementary book or chapter upon the eye, but for the purpose of explaining, the exercises I practice, this information should be sufficient.

As I lie in bed I look far to the right, then far to the left, then close the eyes tightly as possible several times. Then, with eyes opened, turn them from obliquely upward to the right to obliquely downward to the left. Variation—roll eyes in a wide circle to the right; look far upward then far downward; turn eyes from obliquely upward at the left to obliquely downward at the right. Roll eyes in a wide circle to the left. During these exercises I strike both temples rapidly with the heels of my open hands.

This last percussion exercise has a wonderfully invigorating effect upon the eyes and will surely improve the sight. The reason for this is that it draws the blood to them and increases their vitality by enabling them to secure more and better nourishment. It also stimulates the nervous structure of the eyes.

In commencing these exercises great care should be taken not to overdo them and for the first few times "go slow." I practice them now only in the morning as I lie in bed and afterwards I douche the eyes at the water faucet.

The percussion example for the temples I learned from an old printer who practiced it and the eye-rolling exercises whenever his eyes became tired. His eyes were in excellent shape and he informed me that he often practiced both exercises during his work with great benefit.

Bernarr Macfadden, editor of The Physical Culture Magazine, of New York, has published an excellent little book entitled "Strong Eyes." The price is one dollar. The percussion exercise is not included in it, but the eye-rolling exercises are and are excellently illustrated. I advise you to get that book and read it carefully. It contains many good suggestions, which space will not permit me to describe.

The best proof of the efficiency of the eye exercise is that now at 72 my sight has improved to such an extent that I have been able to prosecute without any distress the long series of researches and readings which I have found necessary in writing "The Art of Getting Young Again." Undoubtedly, this great improvement in my sight is to a great extent indirectly due to my excellent physical condition, but it is certainly directly due to the practice of the exercises I describe, and I am certain I could not have made this success if I had not systematically and persistently practiced those eye exercises. Therefore, if the muscles of your eyes are weak I advise you to follow my example. You will then surely strengthen them. I would also add if you will strengthen the rest of your body by the methods described in this book you will have no reason to regret following my advice, for this is "How I Strengthened My Eyes."

The Liver

WHEN the liver is wrong everything seems wrong, for the health of the body depends largely upon its condition and activity. If it secretes bile normally, and performs its other functions healthfully, then the whole body has the benefit of its good work; but if, on the other hand, it is lazy or congested, troubles commence; a torpid or fractious liver being a very serious affliction. The list of troubles resultant from this condition is a long one.

The liver is really a filter through which the blood must pass to be purified, and if this process of purification is improperly performed the blood is poisoned, and any or all of the organs may be affected more or less seriously. When the liver is sluggish there is usually a dull, aching pain in the right side, and ofter under the right shoulder blade. Then, too, there are pains in the forehead (more rarely in the back of the head); furred tongue; an unpleasant taste in the mouth at morning; a dingy, yellow color in the whites of the eyes; loss of appetite, and often dizziness; drowsiness after meals, and a generally pessimistic view of life.

These are some of the disagreeable conditions that result, in varying degrees of intensity, and there are others more serious that may follow, if this, one of the most important organs of the human system, is not kept up to its normal activity.

Without going into the physiological details and functions of the liver, think of it simply as a filter through which the blood must pass to be freed from its impurities, and remember that it must be kept in an active state to properly perform its duties. To accomplish this it must be exercised, as must every other organ of the body, the simplest and most effective method being rhythmical agitation, or massage, performed by oneself in bed, preferably in the early morning, when the stomach is empty.

It is best to first acquaint yourself with the position, size, and general characteristics of the liver, before commencing the exercises that follow. The liver is a gland, or rather a multitude of glands, bound together in one conglomerate body. In an adult, it usually weighs four pounds, and is nearly one foot in length in its longest dimension. It is situated upon the right side of the body. It occupies a large space in the abdomen just under the diaphragm, and is partially covered by the lower ribs. The most accessible point for its exercise or agitation is immediately above the angle of the right hip bone, and under the lower ribs.

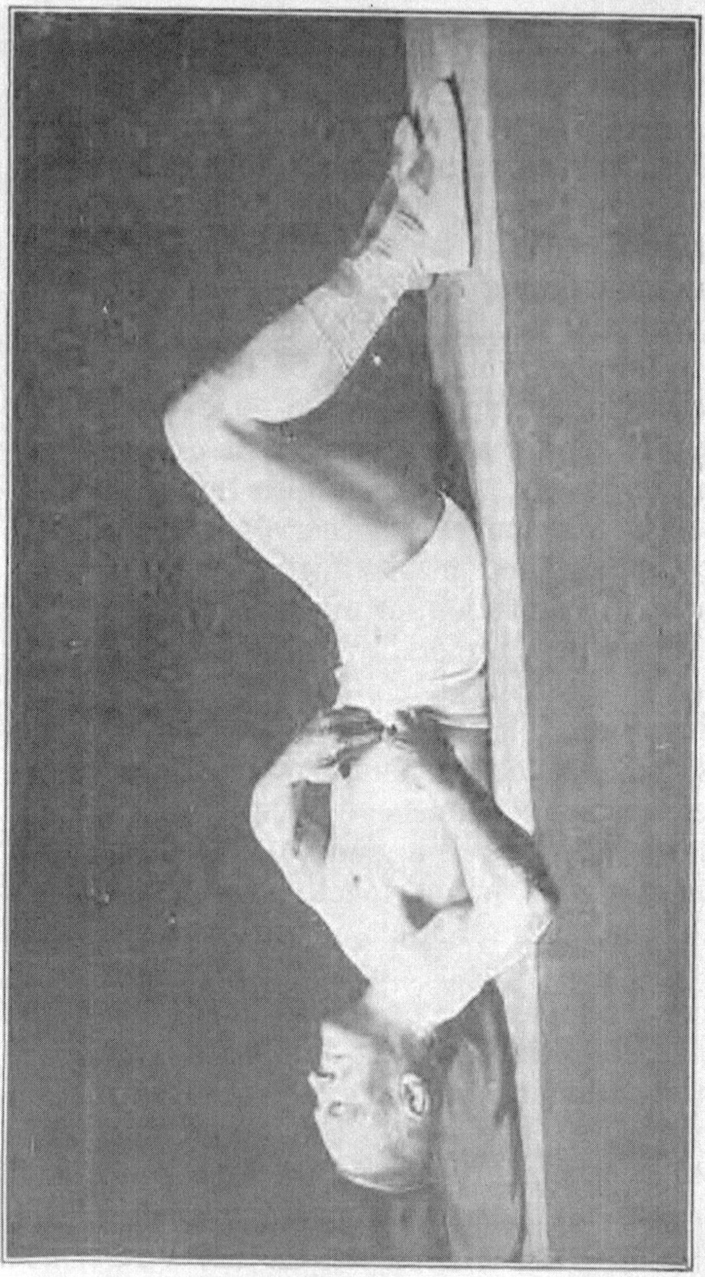

The Liver—First Exercise

It is held firmly in place by five strong ligaments, and nothing but great abuse, such as tight lacing, unnatural pressure, or accidental injury to the region, can displace it; hence there is no possibility that the method of exercise I describe will injure the organ. After five years of practice I can confidently state that benefit alone will result, and that under the most comfortable conditions, and without medicine or expense.

The practice of the three exercises which follow, in combination with those previously described, will surely relieve you of the presence of that child of the Evil One—liver complaint—and its companion—dyspepsia.

First Exercise

Lying on your back, as shown in the illustration on the opposite page, place the ends of the fingers of both hands over that region of the liver at the right side of the abdomen, above the angle of the right hip bone, and below the edge of the lower rib. Then press the fingers upward and well under the rib. The abdominal muscles, being in a relaxed condition in this position, will readily yield to the pressure, and the liver can easily be moved or agitated. Press under and upward, and then relax the pressure, commencing with twenty movements, and in-

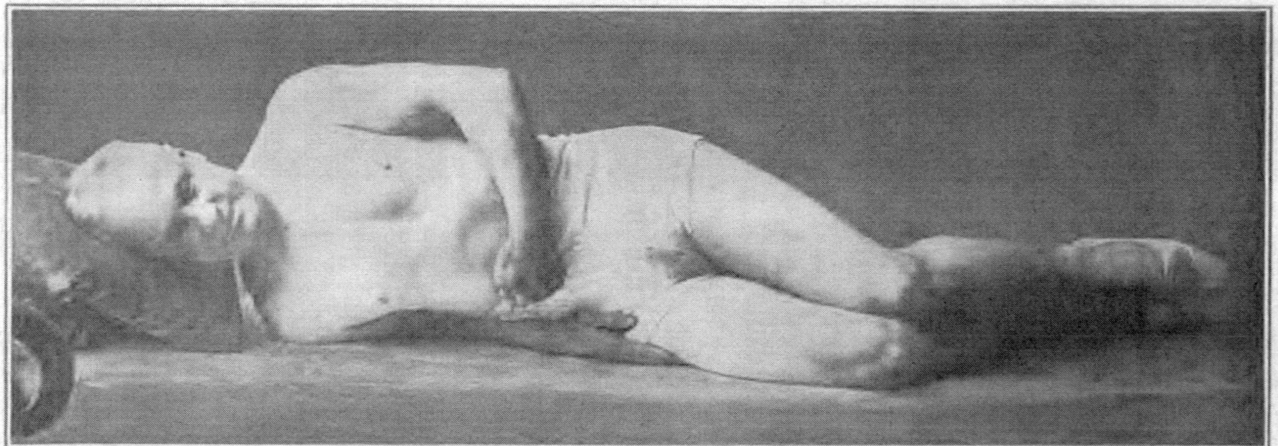

The Liver—Second Exercise

creasing up to one hundred when your condition will warrant.

The effect of this agitation of the organ is the same as that obtained in riding a trotting horse, an exercise universally recommended by physicians when the liver is sluggish.

Second Exercise

Lying upon your right side, place your left hand over the region of the liver previously described. Incline the head slightly forward and bend the knees, as shown in the illustration on the opposite page. (In this position the abdominal muscles will be relaxed and the liver inclined slightly forward.) Press either the ends of the fingers, or the knuckle of the thumb, well under the ribs, and massage, or agitate, the liver as in the preceding exercise.

While it is true that the first exercise may be sufficient, yet this change of position seems to present another surface for manipulation; and both positions can be practiced with good results.

Third Exercise (Percussion)

Percussion over the region of the liver will also promote its activity. The most advantageous position is upon the left side, the organ then being inclined slightly forward, and the

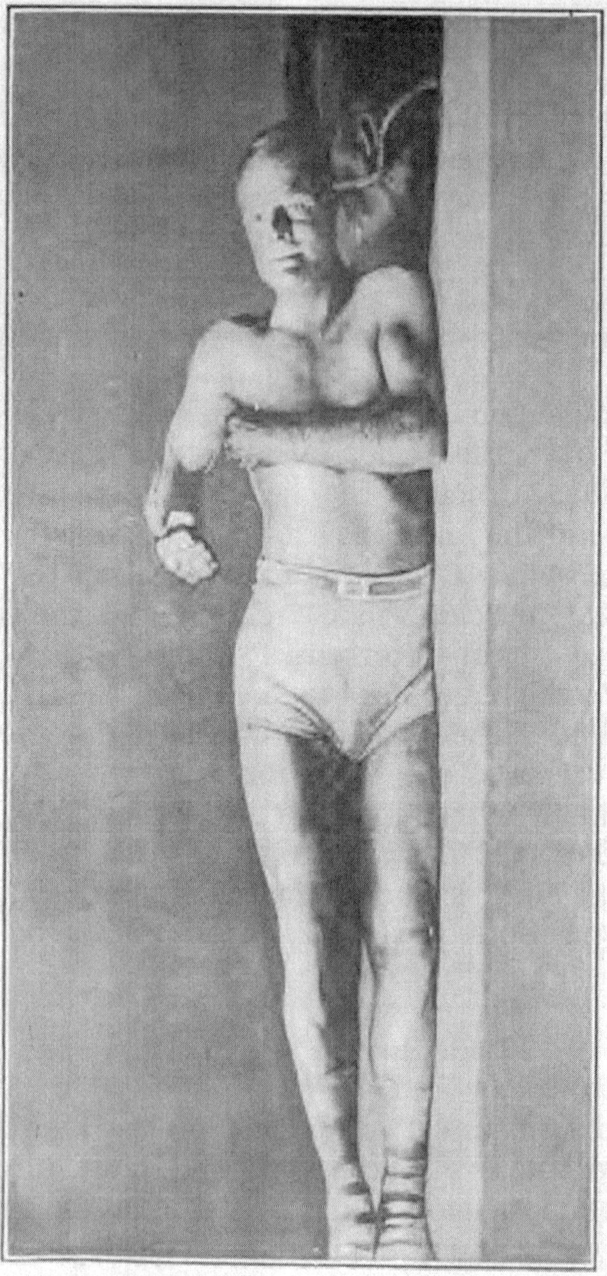

The Liver—Third Exercise

muscles relaxed. Clench the right hand and strike lightly, but rapidly, at the point described.

Commence with twenty light blows, increasing the number to one hundred or more, as your condition will warrant.

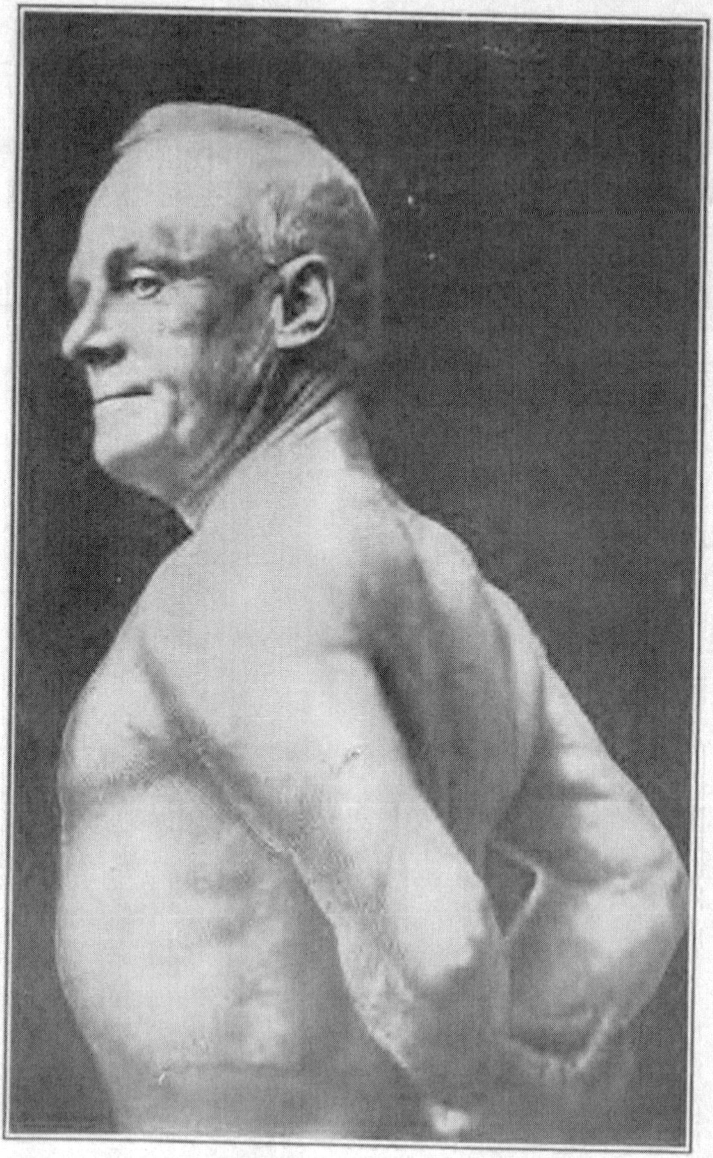

Chest Development, Showing Result of Deep-Breathing Exercise

Deep-Breathing Exercises for the Development of the Lungs

A TREATISE upon the simple exercises and methods by which I am physically a young man at seventy-two would be incomplete without a page upon breathing; for to breathe is to live, and "without breath, there is no life." Differ as we may as to the virtues of the innumerable remedies and systems advocated throughout the world for the preservation of health, we all agree that life is absolutely dependent upon the act of breathing, and that man cannot be healthy unless this function is performed as Nature intended.

At the commencement the infant draws a long, deep breath, instinctively retaining it to extract from the air its life-giving property; then exhales it in a long wail, and its life upon earth begins. At the end, with the chill of death upon him, the heart of the old man flutters faintly—then one gasp—he ceases to breathe, and the life principle, dependent upon that act, leaves the body forever. From the first faint breath of the infant, to the last gasp of the dying man, it is one long story of continued breathing, for life is but a series of breaths.

Man may exist for a month without eating, a much shorter time without drinking, but without breathing his existence upon this earth will be measured by a few—a very few—minutes. "Air is life," and without pure air good health is impossible; therefore keep in the open air as much as possible. See that your home is well ventilated, and sleep with your windows open. As you walk, frequently inhale deeply, filling the lungs slowly as full as possible without any feeling of dizziness, then exhale slowly, allowing the duration of inhalation and exhalation to be about equal. Practice this exercise as much as possible in the sunlight, for we are all dependent upon the sun for the life principle; its rays are filled with vibrations of energy and life, and the air vitalized by sunlight is an inexhaustible storehouse from which we extract the vital force as we breathe.

As you lie in bed in the morning, with the windows open, practice this deep-breathing exercise, the same movement as in walking. The most convenient position is upon your side or back.

It must be admitted that athletes or professional strong men are, as a rule, short lived, consumption and pneumonia being most frequently the cause of death among that class of men who, by reason of their strength and physical development, would seem to be immune from those diseases. Usually the sudden death of a noted athlete from pneumonia is attributed to dissipation after the arduous work of preparation for some athletic event, or undue exertion when "out of training." While this is often the case, it will not account for the deaths, by consumption and pneumonia, of a number of professional strong men, who were noted for their abstemious lives. The real reason has been that their bodies were unequally exercised; the external muscles being developed to their fullest capacity, but the lungs, being neglected, have remained in their original condition, and far inferior in their development to the powerful external structure. In this condition any unusual strain or exposure which might not have any deleterious effect upon the strong and thoroughly seasoned external muscles, might work very serious injury to the comparatively weak and poorly-developed lungs. Like a chain, which is only as strong as its weakest link, this, the weakest part of the body, suffers.

If you would be healthy, develop the body evenly; and if these exercises for the lungs are practiced as described, you need not fear pulmonary diseases.

I speak from experience, for my father died of consumption at the age of forty-two. I inherited weak lungs and a tendency to that dread disease. By these lung-strengthening exercises, I have increased the expansion of my chest from two and one-half inches to five and one-half inches, and am absolutely free from coughs, colds, or any lung weakness. I strongly urge the adoption of these deep-breathing exercises, in this or any other system of training or physical culture.

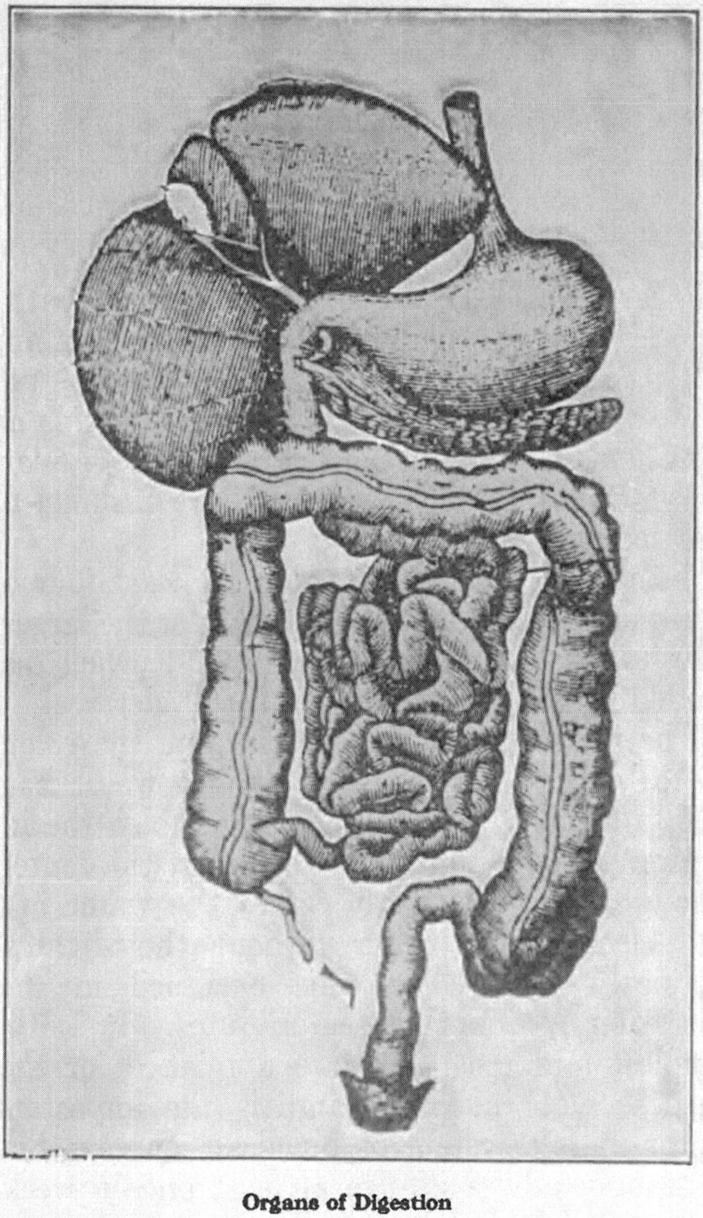

Organs of Digestion

Cleanliness

Internal

I EARNESTLY advise the "internal bath" —what is usually designated as "flushing the colon," or "rectal irrigation"—but most decidedly not what is known as taking an injection. Mere injections of a pint or a quart of water, as usually practiced, are insufficient and ineffective.

To properly wash the colon, at least four or five quarts of water are necessary, for the largest intestine is five feet in length, and when distended is fully three inches in diameter.

The proper appliance for cleaning the colon, or the large intestine, is a rubber water bag, with a capacity of five quarts, to which the injection pipe, or point, is attached at the center. The weight of the body forces the water into and cleanses the colon without the slightest physical effort. The time occupied in this operation is about fifteen minutes. It is the simplest and most effective appliance for this purpose yet invented, and is an important factor in my system of physical rejuvenation. I strongly advise its use at least once a week. It is called "The Cascade," and is for sale by the Tyrrell Hygienic Institute, 1562 Broadway, New York. I cheerfully give the appliance this endorsement in return for the benefits I have derived from its use.

The importance of keeping this large intestine clear of obstruction is easily apparent. It is the receptacle for the waste matter of the system, and may be termed the sewer of the body. If it is allowed to become clogged with fecal matter, as is the case in constipation, it becomes the incubating ground of disease-breeding germs, and the source of all manner of diseases and complications, which would not occur if it were kept properly clean. Physic is but a poor method of attaining the end. The internal bath, by the process described, is the only logical, simple, and effective method by which it can be accomplished. To those who read this book and adopt my system of exercises, I strongly urge its practice, at least once a week, though twice a week is better.

Cleanliness

External

THE skin protects the soft and sensitive parts of the body from mechanical injury, and from the effects of heat or cold. It has over two million sweat tubes, aggregating several miles in length, through which it throws off from ten to fifteen thousand grains of dead matter daily. The under layer of skin is covered with a complete network of blood vessels spreading over a surface of nearly fifteen square feet.

There are also numerous oil glands which constantly throw off fatty secretions; an active, clean, healthy skin is, therefore, a very important factor in the process of eliminating dead and clogging matter, and in greatly aiding the work of the kidneys and lungs. It is essentially one of the principal conditions of health, while, on the other hand, an inert, dirty skin must necessarily increase the labor of the organs mentioned, hasten their decay, and shorten life. By profuse sweating the weight of the body, when in a gross condition, and when there exists an excess of adipose tissue, can be reduced from two to five pounds in an hour.

When the skin is in an inert, stagnant condition, any sudden change in the atmosphere, which could have no injurious effect upon a healthy, vigorous skin, may produce a chill by which the secretions are checked, with the result that a large amount of blood may be driven to the interior and some of the organs may become congested. A bad cold, with all of its attendant discomforts, may follow, with the possibility even of other and more serious complications.

The necessity of keeping the pores open and free, to eliminate the waste matter, is quite evident, and the very best way to remove the surface dirt and accomplish the desired end is by the plentiful and frequent use of soap and warm water. Previous to the bath, create a friction on the back and shoulders and back of the legs with a rough Turkish towel, and on the chest, stomach and front of the legs with horse-hair mittens, which can be purchased at almost any drug store. This will loosen the dead epidermic scales and the impurities lodged upon the skin, and greatly add to the benefit of the bath.

I advise the tepid bath; it is very true there is usually an invigorating effect in the cold bath where prompt reaction follows, but in the case of persons of advanced years, or those in poor health, recovery from the shock of cold water may not be prompt, and a distinct lowering of the vital force will temporarily follow. The face will appear drawn, and a sensation of exhaustion will be felt for some time afterwards; while, with the tepid bath, if the skin is previously subjected to vigorous friction—as described—the circulation will be accelerated, and the same tonic effect will be obtained, without any lowering of the nervous energy.

The water should be of about the same temperature as the skin. If it be too hot, and the bath prolonged, the muscles will relax, and a feeling of lassitude will result. Therefore, my advice to those advanced in years, or in poor health, is to use the tepid bath as the "happy medium." Create a friction on the body as directed; then let there be a quick, but total, immersion. This practice daily will be sufficient to keep the skin in a healthy condition.

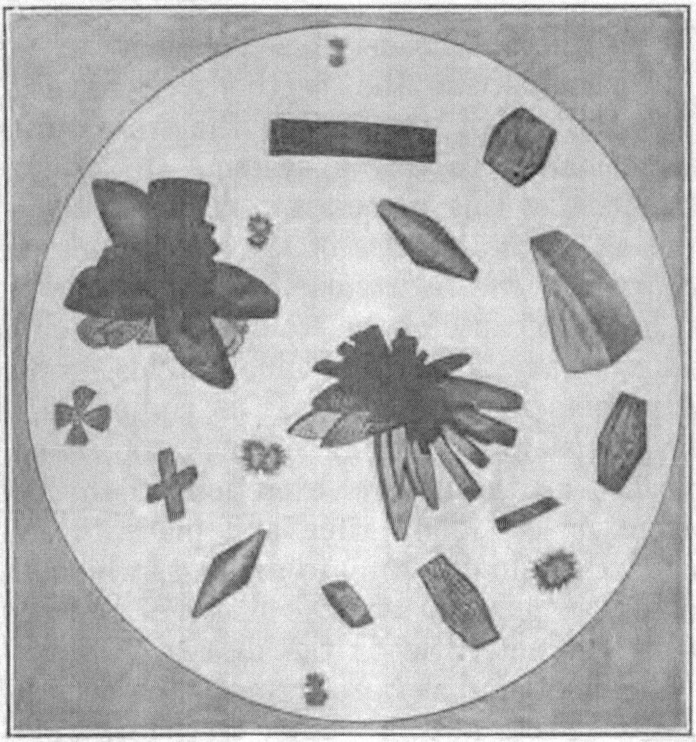

Uric Acid Crystals

Rheumatism

TO those who have a tendency to acid rheumatism the methods I have described of eliminating the worn-out, or dead, matter from the system, are of great benefit. By this process of systematically exercising *all the muscles of the body by alternate contractions and relaxations*, the uric acid which is the basic cause of the trouble, and which the kidneys have failed to eliminate, finds no place of permanent lodgment. It is compelled, by the persistent agitation, to "move on," and is expelled by the natural excretions of the body before it has found time and place to settle and form into the minute crystals, which, like so many splinters, are the cause of the acute pains characteristic of the disease.

Rheumatism has been termed "the disease of age." This is not altogether true, for, while it must be admitted, that as we advance in years it is ever to be dreaded, to think that it is the inevitable disease of age is an error. It should be termed, rather, the disease of inaction and consequently disordered digestion.

The remedy is systematic muscular activity. In this way it is possible to eliminate from the system the cause of the disease. The simplest, most effective and easiest method is described in these pages. I know from my own experience, and the experience of those who have followed my example, that this system of exercising every muscle of the body will surely prevent this most painful ailment; and, when it is not too far advanced, will effect a cure which may not be possible by the drug method.

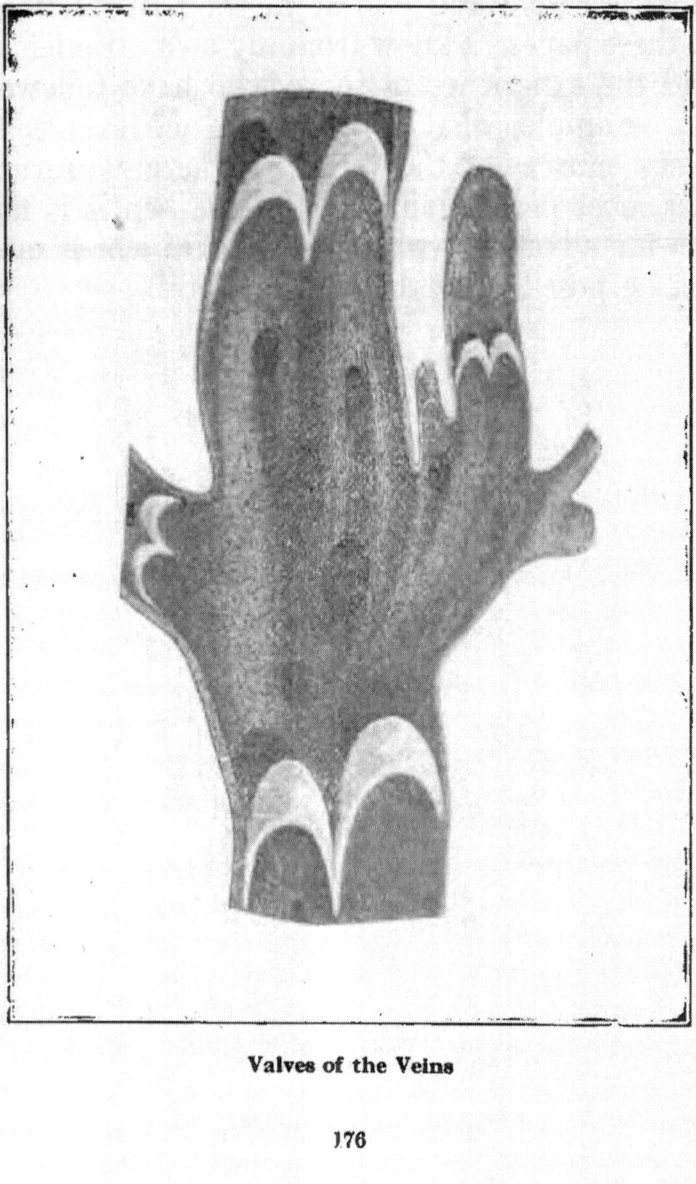

Valves of the Veins

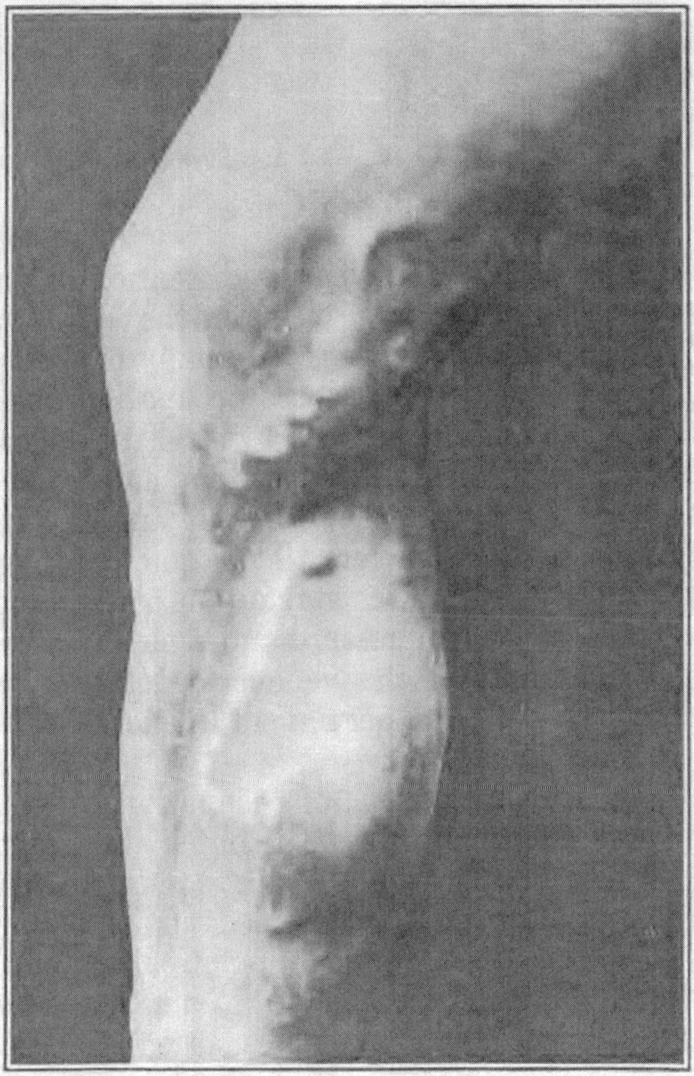

Varicose Veins

Varicose Veins in the Legs—the Cause and the Cure

AS we advance in years a distention of portions of the large veins in the legs is apt to appear. This is especially noticeable in the case of persons whose occupation necessitates a standing position, with little chance for exercise. Clerks, bookkeepers, and workers at "the bench" in the different trades principally are the sufferers. This quiescent; upright position produces stagnation of the blood in the legs; hence pressure and a steady strain upon the walls of the venous system at that point. Result, a permanent distention, or "varicose veins."

In youth, if a change of occupation is made, this affliction may disappear, but if the trouble ensues in or after middle age a cure by any lotion or other medicinal remedy is impossible.

It is true that a surgical operation will effect a cure, but that method of relief is expensive and painful, and will necessitate a discontinuance of occupation during the healing process. Temporary relief can be obtained by the use of an elastic stocking, but without this support a continuance of the occupation and position which caused the trouble will surely induce its return.

The first indication of a varicose vein is a dull, aching pain. The vein becomes much larger, knotted and distended; in extreme cases a rupture of the wall sometimes follows. This is infrequent, but always possible.

In the clinical report of my physical condition made by Doctor Carl Renz, February 5, 1895, which appears in the first pages of this book, he notes "varicose vein upon the inside of the right leg (uses an elastic stocking)." This affliction is a common one, is always annoying, and, writing from personal experience, often extremely painful.

It appeared when I had reached my fortieth year and annoyed me for eighteen years thereafter. I relieved myself of the trouble by the persistent practice of the simple exercise or method which I shall describe.

But first, to understand this method of cure, it is necessary to acquaint yourself with the structure of the weakened vein. You will then readily comprehend why the exercise I practice and advise is beneficial. The following brief description of the venous system is a summary of a long chapter upon this subject taken from the standard text book—Gray's Anatomy. I have omitted the technical and scientific terms that the description may be readily understood by the average reader.

The veins are the vessels which serve to return the blood from the capillaries of the different parts of the body to the heart. The veins are found in nearly every tissue of the body. They are larger and altogether more numerous than the arteries; hence, the entire capacity of the venous system is much greater than the arterial. The arteries, which are more dense in structure than are the veins, are also stronger, more elastic, and preserve their cylindrical form when empty.

The veins have not this property, and collapse when not filled with blood. They have thinner walls than the arteries and are not so well supplied with muscular fibre; hence they are more liable to distention at any part where stagnation is liable to occur. All of the larger veins are provided with valves. Their shape and position are shown in the illustration on page 176. These valves serve to prevent the reflux of the blood. They are attached by their convex edges to the walls of the veins. Their concave margins are free and directed in the course of the venous current. They lie in close apposition with the wall of the vein as long as the current of blood takes its natural course. If, however, any stagnation or regurgitation occurs, the valves at that place become distorted, their opposed edges are brought into contact, the current is intercepted, and a distention of the wall of the vein ensues, which distention we know as that very painful affliction, a varicose vein.

As the primal cause of the trouble is stagnation of the blood at the point, acceleration of the circulation there would relieve that congestion; and the only way this can be effected is by friction. The most effective method for accomplishing this is with the dry palm of the hand, and the most convenient time and place is the same as in the other exercises I have described—in bed and in the early morning. The conditions are then favorable, as the system is relaxed and will readily respond to intelligently-directed efforts towards its rejuvenation or improvement.

The trouble will most probably appear upon the inside of the leg below the knee, running along the calf of the leg, but it may extend several inches above the knee and along the inside of the thigh. With increased years the congestion or distention of the superficial veins will extend lower down, immediately above and around the ankle. This may become discolored and assume a deep bluish hue because of the stagnant blood.

Relief is obtained by friction, with the palm of the hand, daily and persistently. This exercise will relieve the congestion, strengthen the minute muscles that support the venous walls. and if persisted in systematically and methodically, will finally restore the distorted venou .

valves to their proper position (see the two illustrations on pages 176 and 177), when the trouble will disappear. It is a simple, easy and effective remedy for a very annoying affliction. I speak from personal experience.

The most convenient position is lying upon your side. Commence with twenty strokes of the hand up and down, following the course of the vein, increasing as the skin becomes hardened and accustomed to the friction, to one hundred strokes. If persisted in, a cure is ultimately sure, in any ordinary case.

Concerning Various Methods Proposed to Defer Old Age

ALL prominent writers upon Old Age and methods by which it can be deferred, seem to be agreed as to the principal causes of that condition, but the theories advanced for its prevention are almost as various as the writers, or say as numerous as medicinal remedies advised for a bad cold. Among the few books published upon this subject, De Elie Metchnikoff's work upon "The Prolongation of Life" is best known. The various reasons for physical deterioration are clearly described and the effects of age are well illustrated by numerous interesting pictures. It is the work of a thoughtful, able scientist. But after carefully reading the book it does not seem to me that, aside from the excellent advice to observe certain sound, hygienic rules, with descriptions of rational systems of diet, anything new and valuable is advanced; that is, in the description of the proven methods of materially prolonging life.

To the public generally Professor Metchnikoff is well known as the prophet of the great value of sour milk as a food article. This diet, according to his statement, has the virtue of prolonging human life to extraordinary ages. The corroborating evidence, however, is merely that "M. Grigoroff, a Bulgarian student at Geneva, has been surprised by the number of centenarians to be found in Bulgaria, where sour milk is a staple article of food." Another valuable authority, named Riley, is quoted as follows: "The wandering Arabs of the desert live almost wholly on the milk of camels, fresh or soured, and upon this diet they live two or three hundred years." I presume, from his name, Mr. Riley was another Bulgarian. Anyhow, he seems to have been gifted with a wonderful imagination.

Professor Metchnikoff still further adds to the strength of the evidence he presents by his own statement that: "The fact that so many races make sour milk and use it copiously is an excellent testimony of its usefulness." With a considerable experience in frontier life, and some knowledge of the diet and customs of "cow country" inhabitants, my opinion is that pork and beans would speedily take the place of sour milk in Bulgaria, Egypt or any other country where the opportunity to take their choice was offered those people; that is, if either Riley's wandering two hundred years old Arabs, or M. Grigoroff's "numerous Bulgarian centenarians" could get those articles at the same price and had it. My opinion is that as food is usually scarce in those regions it was probably a case of buttermilk or "belt up."

Professor Metchnikoff cites as a further support of the popularity of sour milk, the Biblical story that when Abraham "entertained the three angels he set before them soured milk and sweet milk and the calf which he had dressed." (Genesis XVIII, 8), the inference being that Abraham knew that even the angels are fond of sour milk.

All this certainly evidences its popularity in countries where food is scarce, but the personal experience of the learned scientist as to the virtue of sour milk in the prolongation of life does not seem to have been very great as he says: "For more than eight years I took as a regular part of my diet soured milk, at first prepared from boiled milk inoculated with a lactic leaven. I am very well pleased with the result and think that my experience has gone long enough to justify my views." Eight years' experience of a sour milk diet might help his digestion, but it is no proof that life can be prolonged two hundred years, or half of that period by such a diet. And outside of that brief personal experience the hearsay evidence presented is not very convincing.

The fact is that sour milk, or buttermilk, in nearly all digestive disorders is really an excellent article of diet, as it is usually easily digested, and usually seems to soothe an irritated stomach.

But this is not always the case. My own personal experience is of such a nature that I speedily abandoned it. Like Louis Cornaro, I only write of my own experience, therefore I am unable to agree with Dr. Metchnikoff that a sour milk or buttermilk diet is the solution of the problem of ages; *i. e.*, the prolongation of life. That it is an excellent article of diet in most digestive disorders I certainly admit, but when you have recovered you will change your menu, and this without much urging. In estimating ages of human beings by their appearance, there is an important factor which should always be considered, and this is that out-of-door or nomadic people, of the type of the races instanced, always look older than they really are, and this would be especially the case in the desert-wandering two hundred years old Arabs of the imaginative Mr. Riley. This would also very probably apply to M. Grigoroff's "numerous Bulgarian centenarians." The reason is that exposure to the elements consequent upon an out-of-door life gives an appearance of age to the face, which years might not warrant. I know this applies to the Ute Indians of mountainous Colorado and New Mexico, and also to the "Horse Indians" of the plains; that is, of Kansas, Texas and Arizona, for I have seen a good deal of those American Arabs, and know that after the age of say fifty it was impossible to accurately judge their ages, and this especially applied to their women.

In making this statement I do not in any way undervalue the advantages of an out-of-door life as a means of longevity, that being my idea of an ideal life, but in the countries where these alleged centenarians are reported to be so numerous, sanitary appliances, cleanliness and all recognized hygienic methods of life are, to quote an Irishman, "noticeable by their absence."

Under these conditions the appearance of age is usual at a period of life which in more civilized environments would not obtain. The errors in age estimates of Mr. Riley and M. Grigoroff can therefore easily be explained. In this country the Mexican race formerly had the credit of producing many centenarians; in fact, if an imaginative space-writer was (or still is) at a loss to locate a centenarian and found that his editor didn't think much of the usual county poorhouse cases, he promptly located his instance of "wonderful longevity" in New Mexico, Arizona, or some part of the country difficult to get at, a significant fact being that with increased traveling facilities and opportunities for other ubiquitous newspaper men to investigate, people in those countries who have lived long past a century are now as hard to find as Dodos. And after the find has been made their age is just as difficult to prove. "Leading the simple life" in a poorhouse seems to be, from newspaper articles, an effective means of reaching the century mark, and from a dietary standpoint alone it sounds reasonable, at least to me, as I agree with Louis Cornaro that we all eat too much and that vastly more people are killed by over-eating than from insufficiency of food. Still, I seem to have found simple but effective methods of conducting my life by which I can enjoy all of the good things I like without physical deterioration, or the necessity of a poorhouse or buttermilk diet.

The gratifying results of my system of acquiring health and prolonging my life are a small-boy appetite and a condition of bodily elasticity such as I never possessed in the best days of my early manhood. When this happy condition is a thing of the past then I will still further experiment with sour milk, onions, garlic and other alleged life-prolonging foods, which have been recommended to me. All of these have had their day of publicity, or short-lived favor, but have then been found wanting in the virtues claimed. Like the hospital cat, I have had all kinds of medicines and health foods tried upon me, and speak as one in authority. In an evil hour an old sea captain induced me to try onions and garlic. I do not know what effect that diet has upon Professor Metchnikoff's leucocytes and phagocytes, but as a means of discouraging book agents or standing off your creditors I heartily recommend it. A diet of onions and garlic may prolong life, but the chances are that something might happen which would warrant the celebrated Irish epitaph: "This monument was erected to the memory of Pat Mulligan who was shot as a mark of respect by his friends." There are a lot more of such fool methods of prolonging life, but the list is too long to enumerate. Health foods are advisable, but I did not acquire my splendid digestion and health by predigested foods, and although I have great faith in a diet which is largely vegetarian, I do not believe that life can be prolonged to extraordinary ages by any particular article of food; that is, per se.

Regarding other presumably logical and to some extent possible methods of life, or by which old age may be deferred, Dr. DeLacy Evans presents in his book "How to Prolong Life" some suggestions which, from a theoretical point of view, seem very plausible, but in the ordinary conditions of life are not generally practicable. For that reason I only partially agree with him. His theory is that "distilled water used as a drink will keep salts already existing in the blood in solution, and therefore prevent their undue deposition in the various organs and structures." He also states that its use favors their elimination by the different excreta "and if the same be the only liquid taken into the system either as a drink or as a medium for the ordinary decoctions of tea, coffee, etc., it will in time tend to remove these earthy compounds which have accumulated in the system."

He also advises fruit as a principal article of diet, giving a list of fruits beneficial, also of food-stuffs containing the smallest percentage of lime, and therefore least likely to form earthy deposits.

In a general way, that is the outline of his system. It is all good and reasonable, but under the ordinary conditions of life nine hundred and ninety-nine people out of a thousand will find it impossible to carry it into practice. As a laboratory experiment unquestionably he is right, but in actual life it will never be generally in vogue. The likes and dislikes of people are to be considered; also the expense and usually the difficulty of practicing any particular system of diet. What the general public want is something easy, inexpensive and effective. Given those conditions, that method of obtaining health and prolonging life cannot help becoming popular.

After we consider all the other systems which have had sufficient publicity or favor to warrant careful consideration, I will describe in detail the simple means by which I have succeeded in accomplishing in my own person that which all the various methods mentioned claimed could be done, but unfortunately their authors failed to prove; that is, their efficiency in their own persons.

Another suggested means of preventing or removing limey sedimentary deposits in the arteries is the use of phosphorus in the water we drink. As this remedy had been endorsed by DeLacy Evans, Dittmar, Liebig and some other lesser scientific lights, I decided to give it a trial. The reasons why it should be of value in deferring old age will be found fully detailed in my friend, Frank Havens', interesting book, "The Possibility of Living Two Hundred Years." The book is a compilation of valuable data in the science of deferring "old age." From the chapter entitled "Phosphorus," I quote "The business of thinking is organic." "Without phosphorus no thought" is a German saying. "Phosphoric acid combines with the alkaline and earthy bases existing in the blood, forming neutral salts. As the amount of phosphoric acid increases, part of the insoluble earthy compounds become superphosphates, which are soluble and circulate again in the blood, and a portion is removed from the system in the liquid excretions. This prevents the accumulation of earthy compounds, the cause of old age, and even removes those already deposited, thereby prolonging life for a lengthened period." The method of introducing phosphorus into the system is described as follows: "Unoxidized phosphorus in syrup glycerine, etc., in doses of one or two drachms, according to the strength of the solution. The alkaline hypophosphites and the dilute phosphoric acid in doses of from ten to twenty drops in a glass of water." I do not know whether the highly scientific gentlemen whom I have mentioned and from whom my friend Havens probably borrowed that idea, ever tried the remedy upon themselves, but I did, and I don't advise any one else to try it. In my case the immediate result was a highly irritated stomach, with abnormal profanity, and it set my teeth on edge to such an extent that I couldn't chew any food tougher than mush for some time afterwards. The fact is that these suggested medicinal remedies for age are almost invariably the result of laboratory experiments. In theory they are logical and should work, but in practice upon the human structure they are hopeless failures. Nature has her own effective methods of cure and also of preventing, or at least, materially deferring the disease, which we term "old age," but she needs no help from medicinal preparations. By studying and adapting those methods to my own case I have succeeded in rejuvenating my old body to a degree far beyond that which I had supposed possible. Follow my example and that success can be yours. While I do not claim that a very bad and chronic case of arteriosclerosis can be absolutely cured by the exercises I describe, I am confident that if when such indications of age first appear muscular contractions or Nature's muscle-pumping method is commenced and practiced systematically and persistently, improvement is certain, and that health conditions generally can be greatly improved, even in my advanced years, is evidenced by several aged correspondents who have written me to that effect. As their ages range from sixty-five up to seventy-six years, the period when gentle muscular activity, such as I describe, ceases to be beneficial is too indefinite to be positively stated.

Dr. Osler created a world-wide sensation some years ago by stating that after human beings had reached the age of sixty they should be subjects for chloroform. I do not know the learned scientist's age or physical condition, but if that statement was based upon his own personal experience, and was the result of his professional methods of prolonging life, he made a sad mistake, not alone in his own case, but it has discouraged and has been a great detriment to thousands of others whose ages approximated that period. It is very unfortunate that such a statement from a prominent member of his profession should have obtained such publicity. Furthermore, it is not true, as at the age of seventy-two I present the physical condition of a trained athlete of half my age, with perfect health, vitality and the bodily elasticity of youth. Therefore, I beg to differ with Dr. Osler, unless, of course, his views apply only to himself.

About the time when, worn-out and disheartened, I commenced the system of exercises which have resulted so fortunately for me, another scientist created a sensation almost equal to that of Dr. Osler's, by stating in a widely-circulated article that it was injurious to actively exercise after the age of thirty-five. The statement of that alleged authority upon this subject was probably also based upon his own life of mental activity and most probably physical inactivity, resulting in an old body. To me it was a most discouraging statement. Still, I persevered and succeeded, and that success has been, as I have stated, far beyond my most sanguine expectations. Nature's law is that: All muscles, all organs grow in size, strength and elasticity when they are properly exercised, and just as certainly, all muscles, all organs, and I may say, every part of the body, including even the roots of the hair, lose those qualities and rapidly deteriorate if they are not exercised. It is Nature's unalterable law. In short, the secret of health and long life is exercise, exercise persistent and methodical, from the time you toddle across the floor as an infant, until the shadow falls, and the vital cord that connects you with the great reservoir of the life principle snaps and you step into the great mystery beyond.

The most perfect man, possessed of the strongest body the world has ever seen, will surely deteriorate if he does not exercise. This applies to every human being of either sex or whatever age. There is no exception to the law, and if you would be healthy and prolong your stay upon this earth you must work for it. There is no other successful method. Diet as you will, stuff yourself with health foods, saturate your system with the most widely-advertised medicinal preparations for the attainment of health, strength, activity and longevity, you will not succeed unless you keep your body clear of all dead and clogging matter, and this can only be accomplished through Nature's method. There is no substitute. There can be none. For the encouragement of those who have reached or passed middle life and think they are too old, remember that I commenced my experiments upon this art of physical rejuvenation at fifty, an age when such improvement as I have obtained was thought impossible, and in the instances cited of the aged people who have sent me testimony of their improvement, the system of exercises they practice and which I have devised was only taken up during the past three years. And you, too, if not hopelessly wrong organically, will also succeed; that is, if you follow my instructions, and you will most probably succeed far more rapidly than I have done, for of the many years I have spent in perfecting the art of getting young again, a considerable number have been records of disheartening failures, wrong methods, misplaced confidence in the judgment of others, and much time lost in the investigation of mistaken but much lauded medicinal or dietary remedies. You will, therefore, profit by my mistakes.

I have now adopted and practice only those methods which after careful trial have proven beneficial and effectual in my own case, and as I do not differ in my physical make-up from other men, I know that the means by which I have succeeded will be successful with you.

You know the benefits of exercise, but the general impression is that it means joining a gymnasium, or performing a variety of violent motions in your bed-chamber, and probably at unpleasant hours. Naturally, in time they become distasteful and are finally abandoned. Exercise is, of course, simply muscular activity; *i. e.*, the alternate contractions and relaxations of the muscles, and this can be easily effected without mechanical appliances, and in this way is far more easily and effectively performed as you lie comfortably in bed under cover of the bed-clothes. And as these movements are performed slowly there is no necessity of disarranging them.

Remember always that each set of muscles should be exercised slowly and by themselves. Under these conditions there is no strain upon the heart and there need be no great acceleration of the pulse. If you have any curiosity upon that point accustom yourself to test your pulsation and if the exercises are performed as advised you will find I am correct. From the great mass of letters I have received I find that the average age of the writers who have become interested in my simple methods of rejuvenation, seem to come from persons of middle age or those who have commenced to realize that some marks of age have become evident. Regarding those persons, or those between the ages of 35 and 55, it may be of interest to know that the pulse under healthy conditions should run at about 72. But in the early morning, after a quiet night's rest, it will most probably run three to five beats slower, while soon after any activity possibly it will rate along at say from 75 to 80. I find this is the situation in my own case, and as I am physically in the condition of a very healthy man of about forty, my impression is that if you are nearly that age you will find your pulse to be at about the same rate. This statement is made in a general way, as frequently I have found great variations from what seems to be the usual rule, and this even when the subject seems perfectly sound, healthy and conditions normal.

The following table of pulse frequency, compiled by Professor W. F. Porter, may be found interesting as it is the work of an excellent authority upon this subject:

Table of Pulse Frequency

Compiled by Professor W. F. Porter

AGE	BEAT PER MINUTE	AGE	BEAT PER MINUTE	AGE	BEAT PER MINUTE
1	134	13–14	87	30–35	70
1–2	111	14–15	82	35–40	72
2–3	108	15–16	83	40–45	72
3–4	108	16–17	80	45–50	72
4–5	103	17–18	76	50–55	72
5–6	98	18–19	77	55–60	75
6–7	93	19–20	74	60–65	73
7–8	94	20–21	71	65–70	75
8–9	89	21–22	71	70–75	75
9–10	91	22–23	70	75–80	72
10–11	87	23–24	71	80 & over	79
11–12	89	24–25	72		
12–13	88	25–30	72		

I am often asked if I smoke. I must admit, sometimes, and I think it is a bad practice. The effect of nicotine upon the heart, arterial and nervous system, is bad. It certainly greatly increases the blood pressure and the injurious effects are more speedy than alcohol, although possibly not so lasting. I do not think my post prandial cigar assists my digestion in any degree and if there is any tendency to acidity of the stomach I am confident that it aggravates that condition. Just what effect nicotine has upon the heart you can easily find out by trying the pulse of any inveterate smoker. The uneven beat of the "tobacco heart" will at once be evident and it is certain that any marked variation from steady rhythm of normal, healthy pulsation indicates a weakening at life's central station. My pulse always runs steadily, but when it fails to do so I will instantly cut out that one post prandial cigar as that will probably be the cause of the trouble. In short, I think smoking is a bad and injurious habit. It is almost as bad as having an interest in a cocktail route.

I am often asked if it is possible in age to restore by any exercise, the coloring pigment of the hair. That is an experiment which I am now making. This idea was suggested by reading "Old Age Deferred," by Arnold Lorand, M.D., of Carlsbad, Austria, and published by F. A. Davis Company of Philadelphia. His treatment of the interesting subject upon which he writes is based principally upon entirely novel lines. Aside from presenting a great deal of excellent advice in the direction of the necessity of observance of proven hygienic laws, general rules for the maintenance of health and the conduct of life generally, he advances the theory that the secret of a long life lies principally in preserving a healthy condition of the thyroid gland. That is the large gland that is situated at the lower part of the throat. It consists of two lobes lying upon both sides of the wind pipe or trachea, below the Adam's apple and at about the third ring of the trachea. In man these two lobes are connected by a narrow isthmus. In woman three lobes appear. Dr. Lorand claims that upon the condition of this thyroid gland our health or ill health and term of life are largely dependent.

As this theory is exhaustingly argued through a work of 458 pages, it is impossible for me to devote in this smaller book a great deal of space in recounting the reasons he advances. After hunting up and reading a good many articles on this gland and its functions, my opinion is that the learned scientist seems to be better informed upon the subject, or at least has written more extensively upon it than any other authority I have yet consulted. This much I have arrived at, that its real functions are not yet wholly understood by anyone. Scientific literature on old age is very scarce, and specific, reliable information upon the thyroid gland is even more difficult to find. That general, healthy activity of the entire glandular system is the sine qua non of health, and therefore probably a long life is evident, but that those conditions are dependable upon any particular gland is doubtful. Still, as every organ of the body has a special duty to perform it may be that aside from being a factor in our general health, one of the functions of the thyroid gland is to secrete the coloring pigment of the hair. Dr. Lorand does not positively make this statement, but intimates its probability.

After three months' practice in stimulating this gland by massage combined with the throat muscle exercises (see chart) I found that my hair became much darker in patches and stripes, but after discontinuing the exercise for two weeks the color disappeared. I then commenced again and in about a week more nearly the same results were obtained.

Whether degeneration of the thyroid gland is the principal cause of gray hair, as he intimates, and whether the original color can be permanently regained by stimulating it to activity by massage in connection with exercises of the surrounding muscles, is an interesting experiment. If I find that he is right and that exercise is not injurious I will stick to it until I remove the last indications of my age. But if wrong, I will resign myself to the inevitable and go on gray-headed to the end. There is one thing certain, the coloring of the hair must be secreted by some gland and it is just possible that it is the thyroid. If I succeed in my experiments and it is safe for you to try, I shall subsequently have more to say on this subject.

Of other publications of merit upon Old Age and methods of deferring that condition with which I am familiar, the following contain much valuable information: "The Possibility of Living Two Hundred Years," by F. C. Havens; "The Art of Living," by William Kinnear; "The Essays of S. Rowbotham, "How Nature Cures," by Dr. Emmet Densmore; "Health by Good Living," by W. W. Hall, M.D.; "The Book of the Ralston Health Club," and "The Science of Health," by Edward Hooker Dewey, M.D.

There are, of course, many more and probably very good ones, but space will not admit of a prolongation of the list; but after reading those named, as well as the views of a great many other recognized authorities upon the subject, it seems strange that so little importance is attached to muscular activity as a means of accomplishing that which the whole world is seeking. In all ages mankind has vainly endeavored to restore to the aged human structure by medicinal means the elasticity, strength and vitality characteristic of youth. This has been the disappointed dream of the early alchemist and it is still the faint, wavering hope of science, but as years roll on with the precedent of countless millions of failures and not one authenticated success, that hope is becoming fainter and with thinking people, the doubt stronger. Still the great mass blunder on as credulous now of the alleged curative virtues of any widely-advertised medical preparation as they were in the century when Dr. Paracelsus and the other charlatan, Cagliostro, excited all Europe by claiming that they had discovered medicinal preparations (they called them elixirs in those days), by which life could be prolonged indefinitely. At least that was the claim made by Dr. Paracelsus, the quack. Cagliostro was more modest, his "red-elixir" only prolonged life to three hundred years.

After them came Ponce de Leon and his fountain of youth. Now we laugh at the credulity of their dupes and then buy at the modern fountains of youth, our drug stores, medical concoctions which, according to the advertisements, cure all the evils flesh is heir to. Barnum was right, people like to be humbugged. It is all very illogical, as if health, strength and elasticity of body and a long life could be purchased at a drug store or obtained by any medical prescription; then the financially richest man would be most generously endowed with these, the greatest natural riches in the world, by reason, of course, of his purchasing powers, and the position of drug clerks who had these remedies for sale would be at a premium, for they would have cures for all the evils "flesh is heir to" at their elbows and presumably at cost prices.

The doctors who administered these medicines, knowing their great values, would take them themselves, and as a result be shining examples of their efficiency, and if any one of the thousands of hair restorers advertised would perform what is claimed for them our baldest and richest millionaire would grow a head of hair which would make the spirit of Absalom turn green with envy. But what is the actual situation?

The financially richest man is frequently a physical insolvent, and notwithstanding his purchasing powers, often keeping alive upon "the diet of a millionaire," graham crackers and weak tea. And usually neither the doctors who prescribe the medicines, nor the druggist clerks who fill their prescriptions are convincing exhibits of their alleged virtues. Manifestly there is something wrong in such a system, and I predict that before the end of the century the allopathic medicinal methods from which I suffered from babyhood until I had reached the half century mark (and commenced to think) will be a thing of the past. The methods of the physician of the future, say in about one hundred years, will be a distinct departure from those which are now in vogue. He will know more of psycho-therapeutics and avail himself of its possibilities. He will understand how Nature cures and will know enough not to hinder that process with medicinal dosings, and after a few thousand more cases like mine (of physical rejuvenation in advanced years) are brought to the attention of the world, the simple, drugless means by which it has been accomplished will become too popular to be overlooked. When that period is reached the methods by which I have obtained this success will be a part of his advice towards regaining health and deferring the approach of old age. But supposing all this may come to pass, what will become of the medical profession? The allopathic "dose 'em as long as they will stand for it" type, the kind who formerly made my life miserable, will gradually disappear; they will meet the fate of the Dodo.

And that fate will be hastened when very probably some day a law will be enacted requiring that all medical prescriptions be written in English or some other understandable language. And when that time comes it is not difficult to predict the finish of the medical Dodo. For without his purposely mystifying Dog Latin prescriptions he would be in the condition of his predecessors, the old-time magician, when shorn of his "black magic" incantations, and the abracadabra, of which medical Dog Latin is the relic.

But the drug interests generally will say, nonsense, it is impossible. Is it? Just remember the great opposition of interested parties to the pure food law, and in spite of that opposition it passed and the prompt stopping of the manufacture and sale of harmful foods resulted. The conditions are not dissimilar. After a long personal experience with harmful medicines administered to me under cover of the Dog Latin prescriptions, and a general feeling of being "mad all over" whenever I think of my experiences, I am not so sure that what I suggest is impossible. There are vast numbers of people who feel just as I do about this matter, and such a bill, if presented to Congress, would have an immense support.

To many this criticism upon mistaken drug-dosing methods may seem to be uncalled for, yet there are very many thousands of such practitioners who still drench and dope their patients with pills, potions and nostrums usually utterly false, and not infrequently very dangerous. They retain the antiquated practices from which I suffered throughout my boyhood, and they will not progress or take heed of the plain, effective and easily comprehended methods by which Nature cures. Nor can they realize that the growing tendency of successful practitioners of the healing art is now to reduce the use of drugs to a minimum, substituting therefor common-sense, rational methods, and by so doing giving Nature a chance. To those non-progressives only this diatribe is directed.

As years roll on drugless practice in the curative art will increase, and ultimately the simple methods by which I have regained my health and physical youth will become more popular with the thinking members of the profession, and when that day comes, instead of my one isolated case of a return to physical youth in advanced years, there will be thousands of such cases. As for the thinking, up-to-date family physician, the man to whom we fly in our physical distress, a good idea would be to do as they are reported to regulate that matter in China. Pay him as long as he keeps you healthy, but promptly veto his bills when you get sick.

I think that system would increase the number of capable members of the profession. Anyhow it would certainly eliminate from it a lot of cases of unconscious cerebration who are simply obstacles to health and longevity.

In taking up the study of drugless methods of obtaining health and deferring old age, you will experience great difficulty in finding reliable text books upon the subject. The list given I have found to be valuable in many respects, but the great defect in all of them is that so little importance seems to be attached to physical culture methods; that is, neglect to emphasize the great benefits to be derived from general and systematic muscular activity. To help remedy that deficiency, I will add to the list of valuable books which I have mentioned, "Bernarr Macfadden's Encyclopedia of Physical Culture." This is a library by itself. It consists of five large and profusely-illustrated volumes. It is a remarkable collection of invaluable information upon fasting, diet, exercise and general proven methods of health without drugs. It should be in the library of every progressive, thinking physician, and my advice to every man or woman who needs such a health advisor is to get that Encyclopedia. In its pages will be found the answer to many questions regarding special matters upon which you may desire information, but which as I only write of my own experiences in getting young again, I might not be able to give you. Therefore, I refer you to that Encyclopedia. It is published by the Physical Culture Publishing Company, and all details regarding it will be found in the advertising columns of the Physical Culture Magazine, Flatiron Building, New York.

The Subconscious Mind, Its Influence Upon the Body, and Why Christian Science Cures

THE question may arise, why should a psychological subject be introduced in a work of this kind? My answer is that the subconscious mind appears to be the immediate directing power not alone of the mechanism of the human body but of the structure of all animal organisms. It is the lowest form of mind or will power and the force which directly controls cellular life; *i. e.*, the millions of living cells which in the aggregate form our bodies. These cells have an instinct to cling together in certain forms, and whether those forms are in the shape of the human body or other forms of animal life, the cellular structure of which they are composed seems to be under the control or regulated by a low order of will force which, for brevity, I will term the subconscious mind. In some of its manifestations it might be termed the instinctive mind, for it would seem to be a part of the instinct to live, the same instinct or lower will, which directs repairs in bodily injuries. Each cell is a life by itself, and as life is but will-power, the aggregation of these millions of cells, all animated by that principle, as a whole must constitute the subconscious mind. When this lower mind or will-power abandons those cells you die and the cellular structure, no longer held together by this controlling force, disintegrates. Above this subconscious mind there is another and superior will or directing power termed the conscious mind; *i. e.*, the thinking mind, the attribute alone of human beings. This is the reasoning power and therefore does not exist in any organism lower than man. This higher mind to a very considerable extent controls the lower or unconscious mind and that in turn influences the mechanism of the body, hence, the power of the human will upon the physical structure, influencing it for good or evil, as it is directed. The old proverb, "As a man thinketh, so is he," is a concise and truthful statement of the matter. If the theories presented are correct, then the reasons why and how Christian Science cures may be clearer and why the knowledge of this psychological law is a factor in the prolongation of human life. It will also explain the necessity of will concentration in the muscle-tension exercises I have devised and described in this book, for by that concentration of the higher will-power, upon any set of muscles exercised, a current of the vital principle is there directed, hence, improvement and growth. The proof of the truth of this statement is that, after twenty years of continuous experimenting in this direction, I find that with will concentration when exercising, improvement of the muscles in size, strength and elasticity is sure and very often rapid, while if there is no concentration the results are not satisfactory. If there is a determination to succeed and persistence in practicing the simple methods described, success will be yours as it has been in my case and also in the cases of thousands of others who have adopted this system, by which I have regained my physical youth at seventy-two.

I will go further than this. I am confident that the causation of the thousands of cures effected by Christian Science can be explained along the lines of the theories presented, cures made in the face of scientific, and alleged scientific, opinions that they could not be effected by such means. Science now explains, or tries to explain, the phenomena under the term, auto-suggestion. It was formerly known as faith-cure and under that name has proved its efficiency in all ages. The king's touch cured scrofula and kindred diseases centuries ago, when kings were in better repute than they are now. Thousands of miraculous cures are to the credit of our Lady of Lourdes, and very probably of many other highly respected saints, faith or auto-suggestion if you will, being at the bottom of it all, and whether that faith relies upon the healing virtues of some dead saint's bones, the laying on of hands, or what not, it is all under the same psychological law. The remarkable cures performed by the simple methods of this new curative science of thought cannot be laughed down. The teachings of scientific schools were and still are opposed to it, but it has come to stay, and cannot be effectually pooh-poohed or laughed down either by real or alleged scientists. The knowledge and practice of this psychological law of healing is as old as the pyramids, but it remained for Mrs. Mary Eddy to popularize it by appealing to the strongest instinct of our nature, the instinct to worship and rely in our distress upon a higher power, the religious sentiment which in all ages has shaped the destinies of this world. It was an inspiration and in linking a well demonstrated curative psychological law to a religious sentiment, she has placed Christian Science upon an enduring basis and it surely has come to stay. Its tenets certainly stand for the moral betterment of mankind, and as years roll on will be a still greater factor than it is now in relieving the world from the stupid medicine habit, and in that way, at least, will materially assist in prolonging human life, which medicines never did. I am not a Christian Scientist, at least from a religious standpoint, but I have investigated the phenomena quite extensively and have had numerous satisfactory demonstrations of the curative effects of this new thought method. I have no desire to steal any of Mrs. Eddy's thunder or in any way to attack Christian Science, for it has my very best wishes; but I suggest that if a rational system of hygienic laws and an equally rational system of exercise for the body (naturally I think my own system is the best) were made a part of Christian Science, human life would surely be prolonged and our stay upon this earth made easier and more pleasant, as such a method of life would make us healthier and therefore happier, better neighbors and better friends. Added to this the implicit confidence that there is a well-demonstrated supreme power which, if appealed to, can and will cure distress, either physical or mental, induces a more placid state of mind, banishes the detrimental worry conditions and therefore is a strong factor in the prolongation of life. These are my reasons for the introduction of this psychological chapter in a work whose object is to show how human life can be prolonged and old age can be deferred. From my investigation of this phenomena it would seem that the fundamental conditions must first be implicit faith that there is a healing power, which if properly invoked, can and will cure or alleviate the physical or mental troubles of the sufferer. Given this receptive and favorable attitude, there must also be upon the part of the patient, absolute confidence in some Christian Science practitioner and the sine qua non upon the part of that practitioner must be absolute confidence in his or her own healing powers. Concentration of the higher or conscious minds of the two parties, both willing that the distress shall be removed, evidently influences the lower subconscious mind of the patient and consequently has often a most extraordinary and beneficial effect upon the disease. The theory I have advanced would seem to be a reasonable explanation of the process and the reason why Christian Science cures. Auto-suggestion is the scientific explanation of the phenomena in question and is a good scientific term, but just what auto-suggestion is and how it affects the bodily structure I have never seen clearly explained, at least without a mass of bewildering scientific terms which are usually somewhat difficult to make clear to the everyday reader in such phraseology, therefore I present my theories free from all technical terms and as I understand the phenomena. Mrs. Eddy happily avoided this difficulty by presenting the matter without logical or scientific explanation, faith, without question, being the foundation of it all. Her adaption of a known psychological law has found great favor under the title of Christian Science and the wonderful cures effected certainly evidence its success, whether it is called auto-suggestion or Christian Science. The tenets of this new thought are based on the teachings of Christ. They are for the betterment of mankind and while I am not a religionist in any sense, I firmly believe that there can be no better or more elevating religion and if scientific hygienic laws be observed, systematic exercise practiced as I advise, and strict observance of the tenets of Christian Science maintained, a prolongation of life will surely result.

Adverse Criticisms of the Author's Statements on Christian Science

After submitting this chapter to a very able surgeon and scientist, who usually looks over my essays before they are published, his opinion so decidedly opposes my views upon this subject that while I have decided to include the essay in this book, I do so with a great deal of curiosity as to how its readers will receive it. Here is what the Doctor says:

"DEAR FRIEND BENNETT:

"I tried to correct your article upon the subject mentioned, but it is impossible from a scientifical, psychological standpoint. It is all wrong, and I advise you as a good friend to eliminate this chapter from your new book."

Now that is not encouraging. Then I sent it to an editorial friend, who often looks over my writings. Here is what he says:

"DEAR BENNETT:

"Your scientific, psychological effort is too much for me, so I turned it over to the scientific expert who reviews such matters for us. He is evidently a good deal interested in your undoubtedly original presentation of the matter, and has sent me a long article, showing conclusively (to his own satisfaction) why you are all wrong and why he is all right. But I must say that after wrestling with an avalanche of mystifying scientific terms, which he has fired at me, I feel as if I had "bats in my belfry" and I don't know any more about it than I did before he explained the matter. I will keep your article for a few days to further investigate, and if any of the scientific authorities I have in mind endorse your views we will use it. The idea seems to be original and 'good stuff,' whether you are right or not. If we use it you will be scalded alive by the Christian Science publications, and then I can hereafter address you as my 'steamed friend.' "

Now this is a cheerful situation, but I will publish the chapter nevertheless, as I would like to know what somebody else thinks of such an explanation of the phenomena in question.

The Duration of Human Life

IN this century in the United States the average life of man is 40.85. This figure is arrived at by taking the expectation of life of the average normal person at the age of 22. This data has been kindly furnished me by the West Coast Life Insurance Company of San Francisco, and being from that source it is undoubtedly correct. But the extreme age to which the human body may attain, or has attained, is an unsettled question. Frequent accounts of men and women passing the century mark by very many years appear in print and are usually accepted without question, but when the statistics of the insurance companies are consulted upon this point a very significant fact is discovered; *i. e.*, no insurance company has ever paid a loss upon the life of a human being who had lived to the age of 100 years. When it is considered how long the system of life insurance has existed, and taking into account the accurate data collected by these companies, the investigator becomes doubtful of centenarian records, and even still more skeptical as to the cases of the two Englishmen who have the credit of having attained the greatest ages recorded, Henry Jenkins, reputed to have died at the age of 169, and Thomas Parr ("old Parr"), 152 years. To any one interested to the extent of hunting up data regarding these cases, and I may add a number of others of lesser celebrity, I refer them to the valuable work of W. J. Thoms, entitled "Longevity of Man," published in London in 1873 by John Murray. The numerous statistics there presented bear evidence of long, careful and impartial investigation of a great many records. It contains verification of a very few instances of human beings who have lived a few years past 100, but the flat contradiction of numerous claims to much greater longevity.

The difficulty of either proving or disproving the date of a centenarian's birth is very great. Naturally the question at once arises, What is the evidence? The requisite would seem to be about as follows: 1st, baptismal certificates; 2d, tombstone inscriptions; 3d, the number of the centenarian's descendants; 4th, the recollections of the centenarians, and 5th, the evidence of old people still living who knew him or her when they themselves were quite young. The certificate of baptism is generally considered to be the best evidence and beyond dispute, but this is almost always wanting or difficult of verification. Every individual who could have borne testimony has passed away, and nothing is left but to trust to his or her statements, with secondary and circumstantial evidence, and this is usually hearsay.

In another old book published in England in 1865, entitled "Man's Age in the World," by an Essex rector, the following records are given: Thomas Parr, A. D. 1635, age 152; Henry Jenkins, A. D. 1670, aged 169; Mary Billinge, A. D. 1863, aged 112, and the Countess of Desmond, 140 years. I will take the case of Mary Billinge first, reported to have reached the age of 112, quoting from a most thorough and exhaustive search published in the London *Times*, 1865. It was demonstrated beyond question that she was born November 6, 1772, and died in 1863, so was but 91 years old at her death. And in the cases of Thomas Parr and Henry Jenkins, after long and careful search, the verdict is that in both cases there is also an uncertainty of evidence. The statement is made that Henry Jenkins, of Ellerton-upon-Swale, a laborer, was born in 1501 and died September 9, 1670. The mass of data is too long to print, but boiled down it amounts to this: It rests upon no better evidence than Jenkins's own statements, and I regret to say that is a rule which usually obtains in the majority of these reported instances of extreme longevity.

In the case of Thomas Parr, known all over

England as "old Parr," he was reported to have been born at Winnington in the parish of Aldersbury, England, and died November 16, 1635, or having, if this record is correct, attained the age of 152 years. Now did he actually live to this age? The facts appear to show that it is largely hearsay based upon his own statements, and there is no verified data to substantiate this.

The same may be said of the Countess of Desmond, reputed to have reached the age of 140 years. The author of "Longevity of Man," after careful research, was unable to verify that record, but did find the date of her death to be A. D. 1604, and her probable age to be 100 years.

In the course of my readings upon this subject I find the following in the writings of a very distinguished investigator and authority upon this subject, Sir George Lewes, of England. I quote his statement: "Limiting ourselves to the time since the Christian era, no person of royal or noble rank whose birth was recorded at the time of the occurrence reached the age of 100 years, and I am not aware that the modern peerage and baronetage books contain any such case resting upon authentic evidence." This does not prove that the duration of life in this apparently favored class is below the average. On the contrary. As an evidence, the Journal of the Statistical

Society of London, under the date of March, 1863, pages 49 to 71, published a long article on the rate of mortality among the families of the English peerage during the nineteenth century. This data showed conclusively that the average mean duration of life among that class is throughout materially greater than that of the general English population. Now, even with the advantage of environment presumably favorable to the prolongation of life, not any member of the nobility had reached 100 years, and in the baronetage there is only one case.

Catherine, daughter of Sir John Eden, Bart., born February 10, 1771, died March 19, 1872; therefore she had lived 101 years. This is the only certain case in that class of favored English life reaching and passing the century mark. Referring again to the records of English life assurance, the policies paid upon the greatest ages are: The Pelican Life Assurance Company, one case at 97; Royal Exchange, one at 97; the Amicable, one at 97; Equitable, one at 95; Albion, one at 95; Rock, one at 94; Imperial, one at 94; Union, one at 94; Atlas, one at 92; Law, one at 92; Sun, one at 92; and London, one at 90. But there is no record of any policy having been paid upon any life at 100 years.

And I find after going over the data carefully that from 1670 to 1857 no solitary instance has occurred of a person who had insured his life attaining a greater age than 97 years. Another significant fact is developed that most of the cases of reputed centenarians are inmates of some charitable institution or people of another race, not readily located, and lacking authentic credentials of their great age. These are a few of the stumbling blocks which the investigator in this field, endeavoring to prove that human beings can live beyond a hundred years, encounters. The question is one of interest to all, but when the mass of data which the writer has looked up for the past five years is summarized, this is the result: The human body does not retain the vital principle beyond 100 years, except in the very rarest cases, and then but for one or two years past the century limit. I wish to believe that man has lived to 152 and 169 years, as claimed by various writers who cite the cases of Thomas Parr and Henry Jenkins, but all data collected flatly contradicts those statements.

Believers in the literal truth of the Bible will probably instance the records of Methuselah, 969 years; Abraham, 175, and Isaac 180, as proving that man in Biblical times lived to a much greater age than now. This is doubtful. Jesus, the son of Sirach, said, "The number of a man's days are at the most an hundred years," giving evidence of what was believed to be the limit of human life in his day. And in the words of the Psalmist, "The days of our age are three score years and ten, and though men be so strong that they come to four score years, yet is their strength then but labor and sorrow so soon passeth it away and we are gone."

Here we have unmistakable testimony as to what was then believed to be the average duration of human life, and what was true as to the number of our days upon the earth when those words were written the centuries which have since elapsed have not changed. While the general average of life, according to insurance tables, has been prolonged under favorable circumstances, three score years and ten is still the average, and 100 years the extreme age of man.

The claim that Methuselah lived to the age of 969 years is explainable only by the hypothesis that the method of reckoning time then was the same as that of all primitive people who reckon by moons, just as our Indians still do. Under this system Methuselah's age reduced to moons or lunar months would be one-twelfth of 969, or say about 80 years, which is probably correct, the conditions of life in those days not being conducive to great age.

The next progressive stage in the marking of time was most probably the discovery of the equinoxes in spring and autumn, when day and night are exactly of the same length. This assumption being correct would give five months of thirty days each, and upon this basis of a year of 150 days, Abraham's 175 years would be cut down to 72, and Isaac's 180 to 74. In this way alone could these extraordinary ages be explained. No organic or structural change has taken place in the human body, as shown in mummies and other anatomical relics of past centuries, which would account for the enormous difference in the duration of human life claimed in Biblical times and as it now exists, and certainly the dietary and sanitary conditions, as well as our greater knowledge of hygienic laws, have made the possibilities for the prolongation of human life much more favorable in this age than they were when those Biblical characters lived.

The question naturally rises, is it possible to generally prolong the life of man; that is, to add one-quarter or even a greater percentage of years to its present apparent limitations? If the cause of physical deterioration can be removed or prevented this would seem possible. First, I will again present the cause of physical age as outlined in the opening chapters of this book. It is simply the clogging up of the arteries, the venous system, and their capillaries with worn-out cells and calcareous matter; *i. e.*, the debris and ash resultant of the process of life. If this system of tubing, which is really the plumbing of the body, can be kept free from clogging matter, that body will remain young, and even after physical age has appeared, physical rejuvenation is possible even at three score years and ten, as demonstrated in my own person. "For a man is surely as old only as his arteries," and my arteries and tissues are now young.

As the tubes of a boiler become clogged up and incapacitated by deposits of calcareous matter, so do the arteries and veins of the human body. Free them from those clogging deposits and it is possible to prolong life past that period which we now assume to be its limitation.

A correct system of diet will aid the digestive organs, and temperate habits in all directions are conducive to health and longevity, but still if there is a lack of general muscular activity by which the ashes of the system are expelled from the body, life cannot be materially prolonged.

The systematic alternate contraction and relaxation of the muscles, as described at length in this book, mechanically forces out this clogging matter into the avenues for its elimination, from which it is expelled from the body by the natural processes of excretion, and in no other way can this be accomplished. This is not a matter of theory without proof, as I have demonstrated its truth by actual practice and success in the rejuvenation of my own body long before I had learned the reason why. But this system of expelling the clogging debris or ashes must be general and complete, for as well may you clean one part of a watch, leaving the rest dirty, and then expect that it will keep good time under those conditions, as to cleanse one-half of the muscular system, leaving the others equally important clogged up. For that reason this method of exercising is designed for the purpose, and does exercise every large muscle of the body, and indirectly bringing all organs into activity, thereby insuring the greatest riches the world can offer—health.

By persistent practice upon the lines as described I have accomplished my physical rejuvenation at threescore years and ten, and by it, if no accident shall occur, I confidently expect to verify the truth of the statement of Jesus, the son of Sirach, "The number of a man's days are at most an hundred years." And why, if the process of repair and elimination can be kept upon an equilibrium, is it not possible to live to double that age? My answer is wholly illogical and without explanation: Because there seems to be an occult law preventing such extraordinary longevity of human life. There is no authentic record that it has ever occurred, and it does not seem that it can be. In the economy of the universe certain limitations of our knowledge and possibilities of life seem to be fixed, and beyond that limit we cannot pass. At least, my researches have led me to think so.

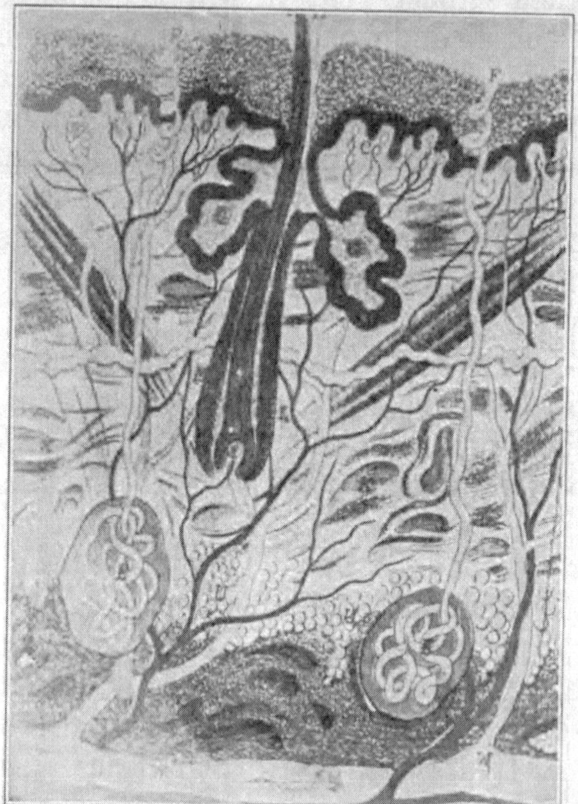

Cross Section of Skin, Showing Hair-Shaft and Attached Muscles

The Hair

TO understand the cause of the loss of hair and how to prevent that misfortune, it is necessary to know how the hair itself is formed, and how nourished, and the conditions favorable or unfavorable to its growth. Having learned this, the methods by which its loss can be arrested, and vitality regained, may be more readily comprehended and successfully practiced.

Facing this page appears an illustration which shows a transverse section of the skin of the scalp. This is taken from a greatly enlarged photograph, showing very clearly how the hair shaft, with its minute muscles and capillaries, appears under the microscope. The illustration exhibits a single hair; it is a tube composed of the same element as the nails or the bones. The secretions by which all three are formed are the same, and they do not appear to decrease as age advances. Therefore the immediate cause of the loss of hair would seem to be, and usually is, local. Tight or heavy hats, dissipation, sexual excesses, weakness of the muscles which are attached to each root of hair, defective circulation, uncleanliness of the scalp, microbes or germ diseases in the scalp, and failure to remove dead hairs which impede the growth of new ones; any of these may produce baldness. Remove the cause, or causes; follow the simple directions contained in this chapter; and whereever life remains in the follicles, or hair roots, new hairs will sprout. But if life has departed from them no power on earth can grow hair.

If the trouble is constitutional, or from any cause which tends to lessen the vital forces, practice the simple system of physical culture I have already described.

The result will surely be an improvement in the general physical condition, and a proportionate improvement in the health of the hair.

The coloring matter is generated in the hair bulb, and from there forced up through the tubular hair shaft. The character of the secretions determines the color of the hair. What the chemical combinations which produce that color are, we do not know; but as years increase, there is evidently a chemical change in the secretions, which causes a loss of the coloring matter. My own experience, and the result of sixteen years' research in this direction is, that it is not possible to restore the color when it has once departed, all of the preparations advertised for that purpose, with the thousands of testimonials to their infallibility, to the contrary. I will modify that statement: you can restore it with dyes, but the deception is sure to be detected sooner or later, and, added to this, the dye will injure the hair.

The scalp is similar to the face or any other part of the body. It is filled with thousands of little pores, which are constantly eliminating refuse matter; in addition to which the sebaceous glands throw off a certain amount of oil which adheres to the scalp. This dirt and animal filth must be removed, or the pores will be clogged—a condition which is very injurious.

When the hair is long, as usually worn by women, the scalp should be thoroughly cleaned at least twice a month; or, if of the ordinary length worn by men, at least twice a week. The best soap for the purpose is that used by barbers for shaving, as it seems least injurious to the skin.

Don't be afraid of water and good soap. Thousands lose their hair through neglecting to shampoo it properly. On the other hand, it is doubtful if any injury can result by the opposite extreme, provided the hair is thoroughly dried after the cleansing process. When dry, a few drops of olive oil will produce an attractive and healthy gloss. The use of hot and cold water, alternating quickly from one application to the other, is of great value as a tonic for both hair and scalp, as it accelerates the circulation of the blood in the parts so treated.

Have the temperature of the heated water as hot as you can bear it, and the other as cold as possible without using ice; hot and cold wet cloths applied alternately is a convenient substitute, if you cannot douse your head with the water itself. The change from hot to cold should be made at least five or six times at each treatment, but double that number will be beneficial and can do no harm. If life still remains in the roots of the hair a healthy growth will usually result. The tonic effect of this process is far more efficacious than any medicinal "hair invigorator" yet invented.

If the scalp is itchy, and there is a suspicion that microbes or germs of disease exist on it, dampen it with a carbolic acid wash. To one pint of water add a sufficient quantity of carbolic acid to produce, when the skin is moistened with the lotion, a very slight sensation of tingling, or heat. This treatment will, with daily applications, require about three weeks. It will surely destroy any germs of disease with which the scalp may be affected. It is an excellent tonic as well as an infallible and clean germicide, harmless, in the proportions advised, and superior to any advertised expensive hair tonic or germicide which you may purchase, but when the itching has ceased, stop.

When the hair is falling out many people are afraid to brush or wash it, fearing a still greater loss, and thinking to retain the dead hairs in the scalp. This is a serious mistake, as those dead hair roots, like any other decaying dead matter, are injurious to the healthy roots near them, and if allowed to remain increase the trouble. They should be removed for the same reason that decayed fruit is removed from its healthy neighbors. Dead and decaying matter is a menace to the life of a hair, just as, upon a larger scale, dead matter and unsanitary conditions are a menace to the life of a human being. In addition to these injurious effects of the dead roots, they impede the growth of new hairs which would spring up in the place of the dead ones, but which cannot do so while the dead roots remain. Remove the dead hairs as soon as possible, and other healthy hairs will replace them, springing from the same follicle, or root sheath.

The process is simple:

As I lie in bed I grasp my hair with my fingers, pulling gently, and changing the position of my hands until every part of the scalp has been treated. I alternate this pulling process by massaging the scalp with the tips of the fingers, which produces a perceptible glow, and has a general tonic effect, as it stimulates the circulation, and evidently determines the elements which feed the hair to the roots. By this hair-pulling process the scalp is lightly raised from the skull. The microscopic muscles and glands thus exercised, and obeying the general law of exercise, increase in size, strength and elasticity, just as the larger muscles of the body are benefited by systematic exercise.

Go without your hat as much as possible. The practice is now popular, being a fashionable fad, and no longer specially noticeable. The sun has a very invigorating effect upon the hair. Baldness, among the races that do not wear hats, is almost unknown; but among the peasants or farmers in southern Germany, who wear their hats or caps day and night, baldness, without regard to age, is the rule rather than the exception. I have lived in an Indian country and I do not remember of ever having seen a bald-headed Indian. That is a hint from Nature.

Many people are afraid to use soap and water upon their hair, and quote self-constituted authorities in support of the statement that their use is injurious. Why should water be bad for the hair of the head but good for the hair of the beard or moustache? Such a contention is not logical, for the hair on the head and the hair on the face are identically the same; and it is certainly a most unusual occurrence for a man's beard to fall out unless caused by some local germ disease. That the beard is luxuriant in some individuals, while the scalp is devoid of hair, is to be accounted for by the fact that such men wash their faces and beard daily, and, in the drying process pull and exercise the roots;

after which they brush it to keep it arranged. In this way they remove the dead hairs. As the skin is kept clean, by the face-washing process, the conditions are favorable to the preservation of the hair upon that part of the head, even though the scalp may be bald.

Another mistaken belief is that when dandruff falls from the scalp it indicates a diseased condition. Dandruff is merely the exfoliation of the scarf, or outer skin, with the dried oil and waste matter thrown off by the glands.

The practice of the methods described will certainly relieve the trouble.

One of the arguments against washing the hair is that it causes or increases dandruff. The fact is, the dandruff was there before the scalp was washed, and the cleansing process merely dislodged it, so that its presence was more apparent.

Perspiration has a very injurious effect upon the hair. Athletes, especially, are sufferers from it, as they usually come in from long runs or other active exercise with the perspiration dripping from their every pore, the hair being as wet as the rest of the body. While particular efforts are made to bathe and cleanse every other part of their bodies, the scalp is neglected, the poisonous dead matter being allowed to remain and dry where it was eliminated. It is this neglect which is often noticeable among those whose excellent physical condition, due to athletic training, would seem to be a guarantee that the poor condition of their hair is not due to constitutional weakness.

Use daily a stiff brush; press the bristles well in; rub back and forth, and from side to side, thus loosening the dead skin, dried oil, etc., before trying to brush them off the head in the usual way.

Have the hair trimmed often; the ends may split if this is neglected. Don't singe it. I do not believe the practice to be injurious, but it is simply a useless and expensive process, which can be better accomplished with the shears. The methods I have described are all logical; they are certainly inexpensive and easily performed, and I know from personal experience they are effective. Practice them as I have done and you need not fear the loss of your hair.

The Reduction of an Obese Abdomen

FAT has been termed the packing of the body; and, while it is necessary to have sufficient of that packing to fill up the interstices of the muscles, thus presenting the roundness of the body and limbs characteristic of health and youth, an excess is undesirable and frequently becomes a very serious affliction. Where there is a tendency to "take on fat" it is usually deposited in greater quantities upon the abdomen than upon any other part of the body, for the reason that the fat, being inert tissue, naturally gravitates to the point of least activity. The legs, arms and back being constantly exercised in the ordinary habits of life, do not offer such a favorable resting place for fat as the abdomen, upon which the deposit will first appear; consequently, in persons of sedentary habits, we frequently find attenuated limbs in marked contrast to an obese abdomen.

To remedy this unsatisfactory condition, various methods of diet are practiced. Of these the well-known systems of Banting and Schwenninger are probably the best. They are published in book form, and anyone interested can obtain them at most book stores. In many cases of corpulence the practice of these methods of diet, if adhered to persistently, will finally effect the desired result; but the danger in them is that the reduction of the system in general often produces a weakened condition which affects the heart. Added to this, the reduction of the fatty tissue, being general, is not especially directed to any particular part of the body, and the discomfort entailed in the practice of the systems does not invite its universal adoption. Furthermore, they involve a great deal of self-denial.

My experience is that the method I practice and describe, in the following pages, is more effective, less troublesome, and without danger.

It is not definitely known what fat really is, or what is its cause. A carbohydrate diet, that is, such as contains starch or sugar in some form, usually produces the trouble; but, when the system has a well-defined tendency to form fat in excess of its normal condition, a course of dieting and attendant self-denial may not always be successful. We frequently hear corpulent people complain that "everything they eat turns to fat," which in a great measure often appears to be true. Fat would seem to be undeveloped tissue, formed in the ordinary process of digestion and assimilation, but upon reaching a certain stage is arrested in its further development, and, instead of becoming living cellular tissue, changes to this inert substance known to physiology as adipose tissue, or fat. When, from some unknown cause, an abnormal tendency has developed, causing an over supply of this form of tissue, it is doubtful if the remedy lies alone in diet.

Muscular activity and agitation at the point of excessive deposit is probably the most direct, surest, easiest and safest method of its elimination. This activity has the same effect upon such deposits as it has upon worn-out and clogging dead tissue, which I have explained can be forced from the point of lodgment by the alternate contraction and relaxation of the muscles. In short, by the exercise I practice and have described, fatty tissue, when thus dislodged, is carried off by the ordinary process of excretion; and my experience has been that, under no circumstances is it possible to convert it into muscular tissue.

Obesity is evidently caused by local inactivity, and that being the case, the only logical and successful remedy would seem to be muscular activity or agitation, where the fatty deposit is situated. Walking is highly recommended and is undoubtedly beneficial; but it is only an indirect means of attacking the trouble, the motion of the legs not especially bringing into action the muscles of the abdomen, which are covered by the fatty deposit. Therefore, some more direct means of forcing into activity, and thereby dislodging this accumulation of inert adipose tissue, would be more effective. It is a logical deduction that, if the fat is accumulated by reason of sluggish surroundings, then any method which changes that condition to one of activity, will remedy the trouble.

The method I have found most effectual is massage while the abdominal muscles are tensed. The process will be more readily comprehended by full instructions which follow.

Fat is really carbon and the phenomena of spontaneous combustion—the cause of many mysterious fires—is a familiar illustration of the method by which fat is consumed in the system and why exercise of the muscles or friction of the fatty deposit will remove it. When the muscles are exercised, that is, alternately contracted and relaxed, or vigorously rubbed, there is an increased flow of blood to that point, and therefore an increase of oxygen, as the red corpuscles of which the blood is composed consist largely of oxygen; these, coming in contact with the carbon or fatty deposit, burn it up. This is the simple explanation of the phenomena. The pumping action of the muscles in their alternate contraction and relaxation expels the ashes, or debris resulting from this combustion, into the venous and glandulous system and it is then carried off by the ordinary excretions of the body. Briefly the remedy for fat is muscular activity, and the exercises described are a safe, easy and effectual cure for it.

Exercises for the Reduction of an Obese Abdomen

TENSE the muscles of the abdomen; place the palms of the hands upon it; press down firmly, and rub the accumulation of fat back and forth, not permitting the hands to slip. Otherwise the skin only will be rubbed, and no benefit results.

Vary this process by striking the abdomen rapidly with your clenched fists, alternately contracting and relaxing the abdominal muscles. The act of contracting is easily accomplished by raising the head.

These exercises are a very effective method of attacking the objectionable deposit, and if systematically and persistently practiced, will certainly achieve satisfactory results. Both of these exercises can be performed most easily and effectively in a recumbent position in bed.

Why adipose tissue disappears under this treatment is explained in the preceding chapter entitled, "The Reduction of an Obese Abdomen."

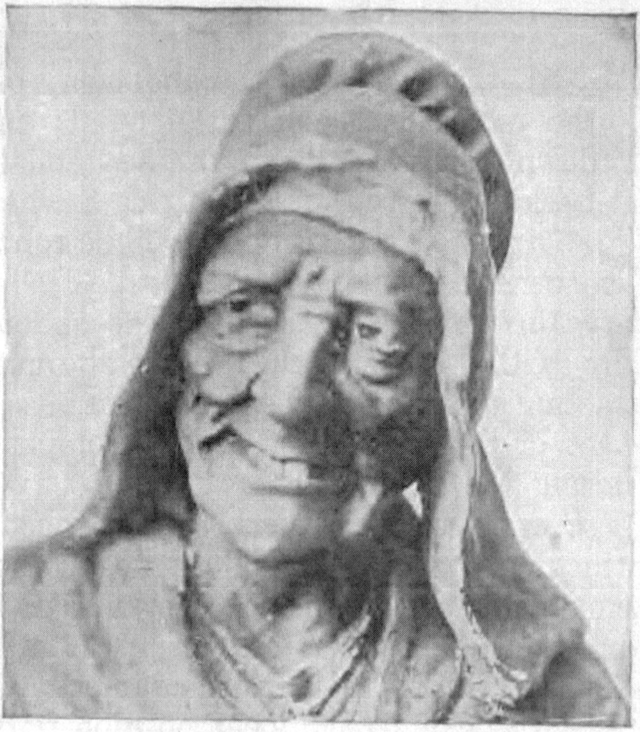

The Flabby Cheeks of Old Age

The Rejuvenation of the Face, Throat and Neck

THE exercises I have described, if persistently and methodically practiced, will surely restore to an aged body much of the lost strength and elasticity of an earlier period of life; for it is possible in this way to restore to the muscles of age the rounded contour they may have once possessed. But if the muscles, especially of the face and neck, are neglected, they will present the relaxed and flabby condition characteristic of old age, even though the rest of the body has been developed to the strength of an athlete. The face and the neck, even while one is in vigorous training, may show the wear and deterioration of years, in marked contrast to the apparently more youthful body.

It is therefore necessary to exercise those muscles just as you have exercised the muscles of the body, and they will surely grow in size, strength and elasticity if so trained. The hollow places in the neck and cheeks can be filled up, the muscles which surround the eyes can be increased in plumpness, and, with a treatment I will now describe, that smoothness of skin characteristic of youth may, to a very considerable extent, be regained.

And this much-to-be-desired condition can be accomplished without cost and without the application of any "skin foods" or other nonsensical preparations of the kind. The process of digestion and assimilation alone can form the cellular tissue of which our bodies are built; and the lanoline, lard, paraffine, etc., which are usually the basis of these so-called "skin foods" are simply smeared on the skin and are not absorbed to any appreciable extent; nor can they be converted into cellular tissue by any amount of rubbing. The skin and muscles, absolutely, cannot be "fed" in that way or with such material, and any improvement in the appearance of the skin which seems to result from their use, is due solely to the friction required in applying the supposed nutriment. If a face ointment is desired, use pure olive oil, or any good face cream; they will soften the outer skin, are cleanly, and, after being rubbed off, will leave it clear and soft.

The true secret of restoring to the skin the smoothness of youth is friction. The skin can be polished and the wrinkles rubbed out like any other piece of leather, and the palms of the hands and the tips of the fingers are the very best tools to use for that purpose. This polishing, wrinkle-removing process can best be done while you lie comfortably in bed, as in that position it is easier, less fatiguing and you can get at the wrinkles more readily when lying down than when either sitting or standing. But before commencing this system of facial rejuvenation it might be well to disabuse yourself of the idea that you can "build up" the muscles of the cheeks, chin, neck and throat or to form living tissue by attempting to "rub in" skin foods. This has been the unquestioning belief and practice of womankind in all ages; (and at the risk of being excommunicated) I will add, at all ages. Of course, my statement that it is impossible will be regarded as rank heresy by every woman who reads this chapter. But when you consider Nature's method of building the human structure, the fallacy of such a proposition must be evident. Every part of the body is composed of millions of infinitesimal living cells (or cellular tissue). These cells are the result of the digestive functions and as this process is only carried on in the stomach and digestive tract, they cannot come into being by any other method, and the idea that the cheeks, throat or neck can be nourished or built up by rubbing in, or attempting to run into the skin and muscles lanoline, paraffine, lard or any of the greasy ingredients which are the basis of "skin foods" is as logical as the "hair seed" industry. At what stage in digestion food is transformed into life we do not know. But we do know that living tissue can only be formed by the digestive process, hence the folly of applying skin food preparations for that purpose—it is an absurdity.

As an advertising scheme the title is an inspiration, but under the light of scientific reasoning it is awful nonsense, and it is impossible that you can build up any part of the human structure by such means.

If the reader is a woman I realize that this attack upon a feminine custom, which is as old as the sphinx, will receive a welcome about as cordial as my opinion upon the drug business; but I sincerely regret to say that I am right. If by rubbing "skin foods" into the skin it is possible to plump up one's cheeks, throat and chin, and in that way generally fix up and make one's self beautiful, a kind of physical millennium would ensue, for all of the skinny people would soon become attractively plump. It is too bad that it don't work, and I am just as sorry as you are. Why it does not can be readily ascertained by reading up on the subject in any standard work upon physiology. Of course, what I say is rank heresy, and I ought to be either fried or scrambled for telling you this unpleasant truth, because pretty much all of you ladies have invested in that kind of merchandise. But it is the unvarnished truth. I found it out long ago by pottering over works upon physiology, and if there is any objection to my statement I will appeal the case to those authorities. But you will say "when I rubbed skin foods upon my face, cheeks and throat it did improve their appearance; my skin was fresher and smoother, and I looked younger." Certainly you did—just for the same reason that the simple friction methods I advise will improve your facial appearance, and if you keep up the practice it will "stay put" and not "wash off." Neither will rain or fogs spoil a complexion obtained in that way.

The reason skin foods thoroughly "rubbed in" give that fresh, smooth look to the skin and why the wrinkles grow less under that process is the result of what is termed in slang "elbow grease"; that is, persistent friction of the skin, and plenty of it, using the palms of the hands and tips of the fingers. In that way you will surely improve your facial appearance.

If after this explanation you still think the benefit lies solely in the "skin foods" which you have made or bought and are endeavoring to "rub in," by all means continue to use them. The direct benefit of the preparation is similar to that derived from the use of axle grease or oil in the operation of machinery—it prevents chafing. Therefore, continue using "skin foods," if you please; they are just as good for that purpose as the very much cheaper articles I suggest, but no better. The benefits of such greasy preparations lie only in their efficiency as lubricants; *i. e.*, in preventing the skin from becoming chafed, in the rubbing process. If they are simply applied to the face or throat without friction no beneficial results will be obtained other than that the grease, etc., will fill up the minute lines and temporarily smooth the surface, but when this coating is washed off the skin will resume its former condition and appearances. This in a way is but a repetition of the matter presented in the chapter upon the skin. But it will bear repeating.

The usual objection made to the friction process I advise is that the skin might loosen and the pores might become enlarged. If you go at it too vigorously that is very possible. But if care is taken it will not happen and even if it did, as soon as the minute muscles and structure of the skin tone up under the stimulating treatment that condition will speedily disappear and improvement will surely result.

In commencing the friction treatment and to keep the skin in place while you rub, stretch the skin with the first and second fingers of one hand and rub with the other, or the palm of the hand. The points which will probably need first attention will be the corners of the eyes, mouth, temples and immediately forward of the ears. To prevent chafing, some lubricant must, of course, be applied at the points you are rubbing—"skin food," if you please, but any smooth face cream will be just as effective.

Don't go at this method of facial rejuvenation

too energetically. If you do you will get sore and discouraged. The same rule applies to massaging the face and throat as to any other system of exercise. Go slow. Stick to it and you will succeed.

Before telling you how to develop the muscles which support the cheeks and round out the chin, jaws and throat, I will give you a "wrinkle" in removing wrinkles, which I think you will find very satisfactory, also very cheap. I have forgotten from whom I stole the idea, but as I have never seen it in any modern beauty book and no one seems to claim it, I will transfer the credit of its discovery to the first female president of the United States. The use of an astringent for toning up or shrinking up the loose skin of age, and in that way removing wrinkles, is a custom also dear to the feminine heart, but the after results are often an unpleasant roughness. There is a far better and more simple way, and it should be practiced after the friction process. To understand the why and the how, I will ask you to remember "grandmother's method" of "bringing a boil to a head." She simply pasted the skin of an egg evenly all over the boil. Inside of a quarter of an hour that egg skin commenced to "draw"; that is, to shrink up and as it contracted the result was a steady, even pressure towards the center. If you have had that experience you will know what I mean without further explanation; also you will agree with me when I say that the only place where the process could be endured with equanimity was upon some other fellow.

The astringent or shrinking process I will describe is upon the same principle. The skin of an egg is of the same nature as the white, the only material difference being that the latter is liquid and when it is dried it, too, becomes a kind of skin. In that drying process it shrinks evenly all over, just as the egg skin did when it was pasted upon the hot, throbbing boil. Apply that process to shrinking up the loose skin or wrinkles of the face, but use the white of the egg, and the same results will be obtained. It is a powerful mechanical astringent. Therefore, instead of the skin of the egg use the liquid white, as I have stated. This apply all over your face, wherever the wrinkles appear, using for convenience a shaving brush. Then let it dry and remain for five minutes, more or less. It is such a strong astringent that it should remain on the skin only a short time, as it may otherwise cause the skin to shrivel. Then rinse it off with pure, warm water. It will readily dissolve and you will be surprised at the smoothness of your skin. If it shines or stings from the contracting process, apply a few drops of face cream, then rub clean, and if you desire, as a final beauty finish, a very little face powder will correct that and give the final artistic touch. This method is good, cheap and effectual, but, as has been stated, should be used with caution.

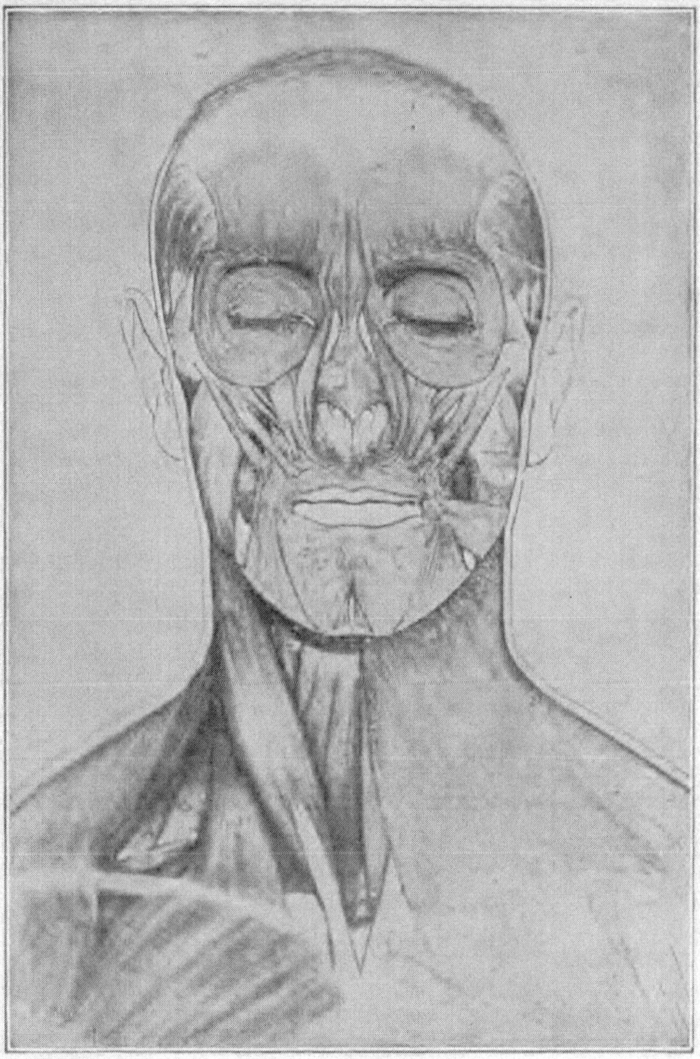

Muscles Surrounding the Eyes

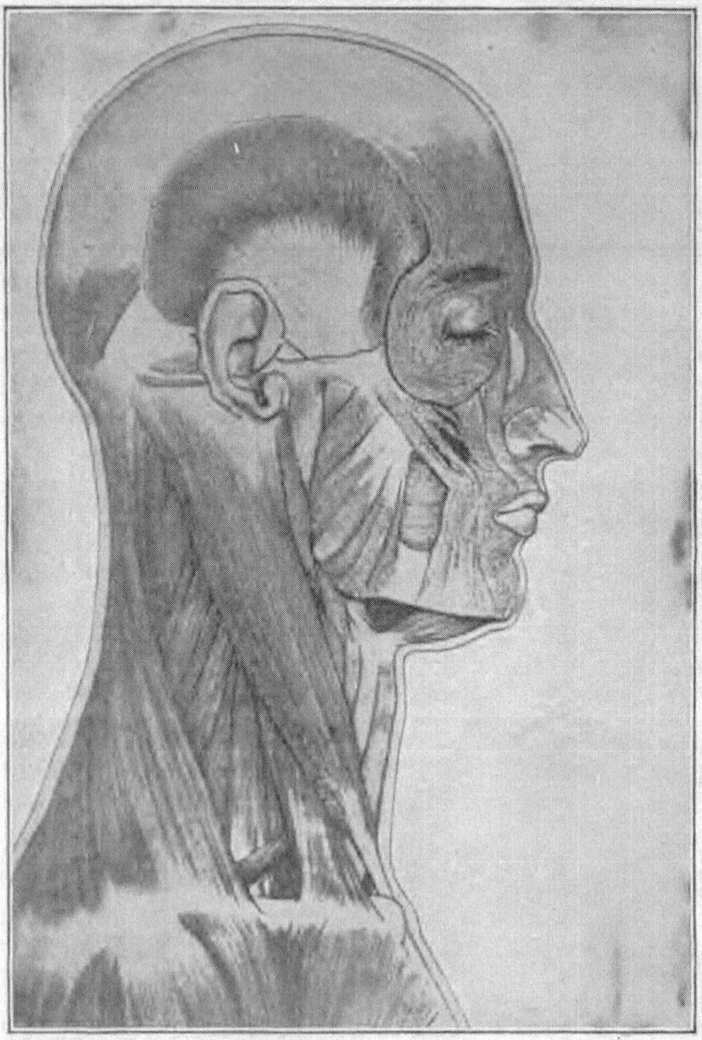

Muscles of the Throat—Relaxed

Developing the Muscles Covering the Chin and Jaws

The Chin

THE cushion of muscles which covers and rounds the chin bone in most cases is involuntary; that is, without practice the muscles are not capable of motion at will. Still they can, to a limited extent, be contracted upward when the teeth are firmly set. This cushion of muscles is under the same law as those supporting the cheeks, and by vigorous massage with the palms of the hands—when thus contracted will soon respond, and if the chin was ever round and full in youth that condition may be regained to a very considerable extent, and this result will be attained much more rapidly than is the case with the cheek muscles. Why this is so is not altogether clear to me, but it is a fact that sluggish, involuntary muscles do respond more quickly to compulsory activity—that is, by firm, deep massage—than those which have been accustomed to activity, either unconsciously or by the direction of the will, probably just as improvement is very much more rapid in the first stages of training for any athletic event than it is later on when the tissues have been "fined down."

As an instance of my success in developing the chin muscles I again refer to the portrait illustration used as the frontispiece of this book, calling attention to the full, round chin there shown, and then ask comparison with the same feature in the photograph taken twenty-two years prior, or at the age of fifty. The full-face anatomical plate upon page 251 will show you the position and character of the chin muscles.

The Jaws

By reference to the anatomical plate, side view of the face and neck muscles, on page 252, you will notice that the jaws are covered by broad, flat, muscular bands, commencing underneath the jaw bone and running upward toward the cheek bones, to which they are attached. The character of the face is very largely dependent upon the shape of the jaws, and if those covering muscles have shrunken, as they usually do in advanced years, the skin will hang loose over them, giving the appearance of age. These jaw muscles readily respond and can be developed by deep massage. This should be practiced along the edge of the jaw bone, using the heel of the hand. This treatment will speedily tone up and increase the size of these muscles, thus giving a rounded and more youthful appearance to the lines of the jaws.

The Muscles of the Cheeks

AS years creep on the cheeks sink in and hollows appear where once they were full and plump. This is due to the shrinking of the supporting muscles, shown in the illustration facing page 253. There are four of these muscles on each side of the face. As we grow older these muscles lose their strength and elasticity, and this change produces the pendant or loose jowl characteristic of age, just as their lessened size is the cause of the hollows in the cheeks. These are voluntary muscles and can be exercised at will, just as you can exercise the muscles of the arms and legs and just as exercise of any part of the body will improve it, so exercise of the muscles of the face will have the same effect. A system or series of movements devised for that purpose has often been described in various essays and books upon the art of becoming beautiful. The method is styled "facial gymnastics, or making faces." It has some merit, and if faithfully and persistently practiced might, to a considerable extent, build up and strengthen the muscles of the face. The objection is that the exercises are very fatiguing and require long practice before satisfactory results can be obtained.

The further objection sometimes advanced is that they may cause new lines. After experimenting a long time with these exercises I have not found this to be the case, and they certainly do strengthen the cheek muscles. But the most serious objection is that progress is too slow for the system ever to become very popular.

A far better and quicker method is a massage system which I have devised and practice while the cheek muscles are contracted. By this satisfactory results can be obtained in a very short time, and with very little trouble.

First familiarize yourself with the position of these cheek muscles. Referring to the anatomical illustration on page 252, you will notice that there are eight long muscles, four on each side. They are attached to the cheek bones immediately below the eyes, from there descending to become attached to the wide muscular band surrounding the mouth. You can contract these cheek muscles at will, this action forming a bunch on the cheek bones under the eyes.

Another very broad and strong muscle underlies these cheek supporting muscles. It, too, is fastened to the cheek bones but, extending downward, is attached along the jaw bone. This may be termed the chewing muscle, and, while it plays an important part in supporting the cheeks and determining their contour, it cannot be contracted or exercised at will, except in the act of chewing. Its action is independent of the cheek muscles, although when they are contracted upward some tension is placed upon it.

In youth these muscles are, or should be, strong, elastic and supporting the tissue and skin overlying them, giving to the cheeks the full, round appearance characteristic of that period of life. As years advance, through lack of exercise they shrink and lose their former size, strength and elasticity, just as any muscle of the body will do under like conditions. The skin covering, then losing its support, falls into the creases and lines we know as wrinkles.

These are the certain indications of physical age, as they tell the tale of the shrunken muscles underlying. For these wrinkles, wasted chin, and hollow cheeks there can be but one cure, and that is the restoration to the supporting muscles of their former plumpness and strength. If this is not done any efforts toward the eradication of the disfiguring lines and attempts to fill up the hollow cheeks will be futile, all alleged remedies in the way of "skin foods," medical preparations, etc., to the contrary.

It is true that by a system of diet, and especially by drinking copiously of milk, an increase of fatty tissues can be obtained. The face under this dietary regime will become more plump and the surface of the skin smoother, but if the underlying muscles are not developed the face will still present a flabby look, the jowl may sag and the appearance of a double chin be more pronounced. These facial indications of physical age are not especially the signs of advanced years, being principally due to lack of exercise of the supporting facial muscles.

During the last five years, or since the publication of my first essays upon the art of physical and facial rejuvenation, I have been constantly experimenting in this direction, hoping to devise some simple, effective and inexpensive method to accomplish this very much desired result, and which could be practiced by one's self. It seemed to me evident that the secret lay in developing the supporting muscles by exercise. The facial gymnastics described did help, but, as stated, I found them much too slow in results.

Facial massage as usually practiced is superficial. It certainly freshens up the skin, but it does not and cannot develop these deep-seated supporting muscles. Muscular activity, directed by your own will, can alone accomplish this. And that is a matter which must be performed by yourself. Here the pauper and the millionaire are upon an equality. No one can exercise for you, nor can any amount of rubbing by an attendant accomplish the beneficial results which may be obtained by your own efforts.

The apparent explanation of the speedy enlargement of the muscles if "deeply massaged" when they are contracted, would seem to be, that the network of blood vessels and myriads of capillaries which thread all structures of the body become distended by blood and lymph forced there when the muscles are contracted and vigorously rubbed, this distension accounting for the rapid but at first temporary increase in size of the muscles so treated. The effect may be termed a healthy congestion, as no evil ever results; and by persistent practice this temporary enlargement becomes permanent, the cheeks then assuming and retaining the full, round appearance characteristic of youth.

I do not claim that large muscles produced by this method indicate great strength, but as a means of speedily filling up the cheeks, rounding out the chin and the muscles covering the jaws, no other method yet devised will at all compare to it in efficiency.

There may be another, or additional cause for the sometimes remarkable and speedy increase in the size of the muscles so treated; that is to say, independent of the effect produced by distending the blood vessels through the forced increase of blood and lymph.

Making Old Faces Young

REJUVENATION of the face and throat is principally dependent upon your success in developing the muscles which underlie, and should support the skin and other covering tissue; for if the supporting muscles are weak, loose and shrunken, then no matter how brilliant the complexion may be, a youthful appearance is impossible and any artificial coloring but emphasizes any "saggy" indications of age.

If those muscles can be developed and strengthened to support the overlying structure as they did in earlier years, then a more youthful appearance will surely result.

This chapter is written for both sexes, and in it I shall briefly describe the methods I practice for the improvement of the skin covering the face and throat, also the underlying supporting muscles.

In the first place, with the exception of a little white vaseline, which I use after shaving, I do not use face cream, "skin foods," powders or face lotions of any kind, as I don't believe in them. In fact the only grease I have ever found which has been of any material benefit in the rejuvenation of my face and throat is what is colloquially termed "elbow grease."

How, then, can sagging muscles be "toned up" and strengthened? And how can hollows be built up? By the same methods you practice when you are endeavoring to develop or "build up" your arms, legs, or any other part of your body—muscular activity; *i. e.,* exercise, is the secret—for all muscles have this property: when they are exercised they will grow and when they are not exercised they will shrink, thus losing their strength and elasticity—then the marks that we know as the indications of age will appear.

Alternately contracting and relaxing the muscles of the arms and legs; *i. e.,* exercising them, will make them increase in size, strength and elasticity and exactly the same thing occurs when you persistently and systematically massage, that is, rub firmly, any muscle of the face.

The skin, like any other piece of leather, is improved by friction, and the very best instruments for polishing it up are the dry palms and fingers. I never use any grease when doing this. Also this friction process will remove the fine superficial lines which commence to appear as we advance in years and when the texture of the skin is therefore not as fine as formerly. But don't in either the friction or massage process do it too vigorously, for if you do you will probably chafe the skin, or by too vigorously massaging the muscles of the face may make them sore—

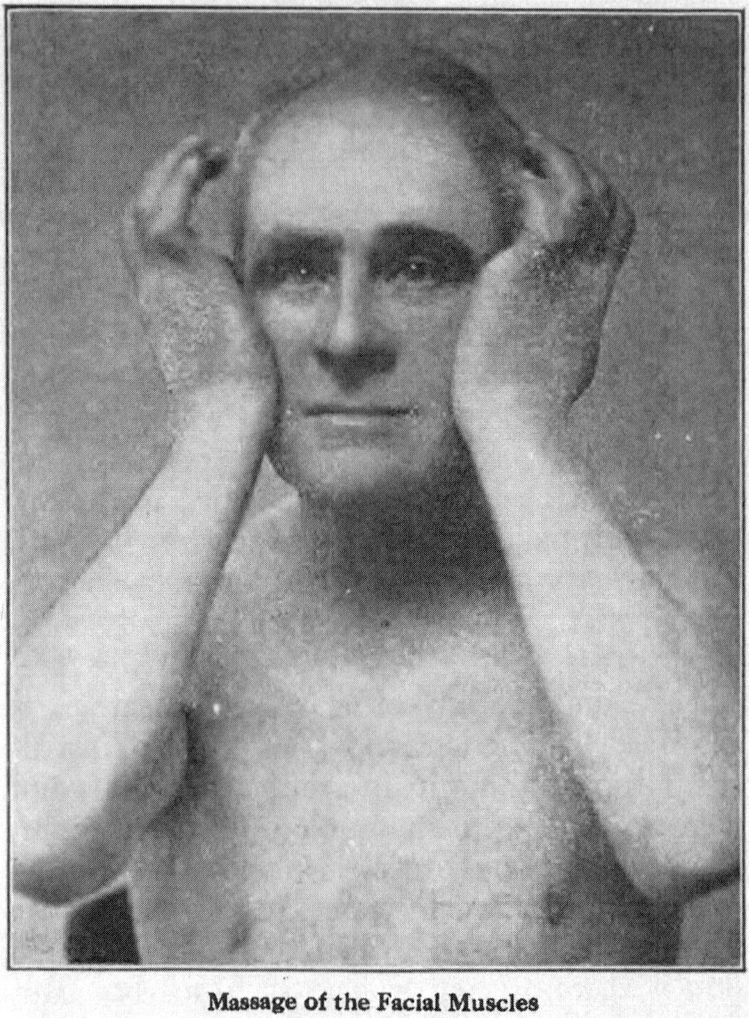

Massage of the Facial Muscles

also you will probably temporarily create new lines, the reason being that there is, or should be, in all faces, an underlying coating of fatty tissue. Now vigorous massage or too vigorous friction will certainly remove this; and until the fat again deposits, new wrinkles will temporarily appear. Such quick removal of the fat may in many faces produce a haggard appearance. This will be but transient, as when the fat again forms, which it will speedily do, the face will resume former conditions very probably with some slight improvement also. Face friction and facial massage are a "good thing," but you can easily overdo it.

The facial and physical characteristics of the thirty thousand men and women who have read "Old Age—Its Cause and Prevention" differ so widely that I cannot provide detailed instructions for every instance, but I have endeavored to cover the ground in a general way in this chapter. If you read it carefully you will find such information in the matter as I can give you.

I will now describe the practices by which my facial rejuvenation has been accomplished.

FRICTION OF THE FACE AND THROAT I have already described, but omitted to say, that the very best and least expensive method of whitening the throat is by friction with the dry palms of the hands and fingers. It is well also to whiten the sides and bridge of the nose by the same method. And after you have finished, wash the

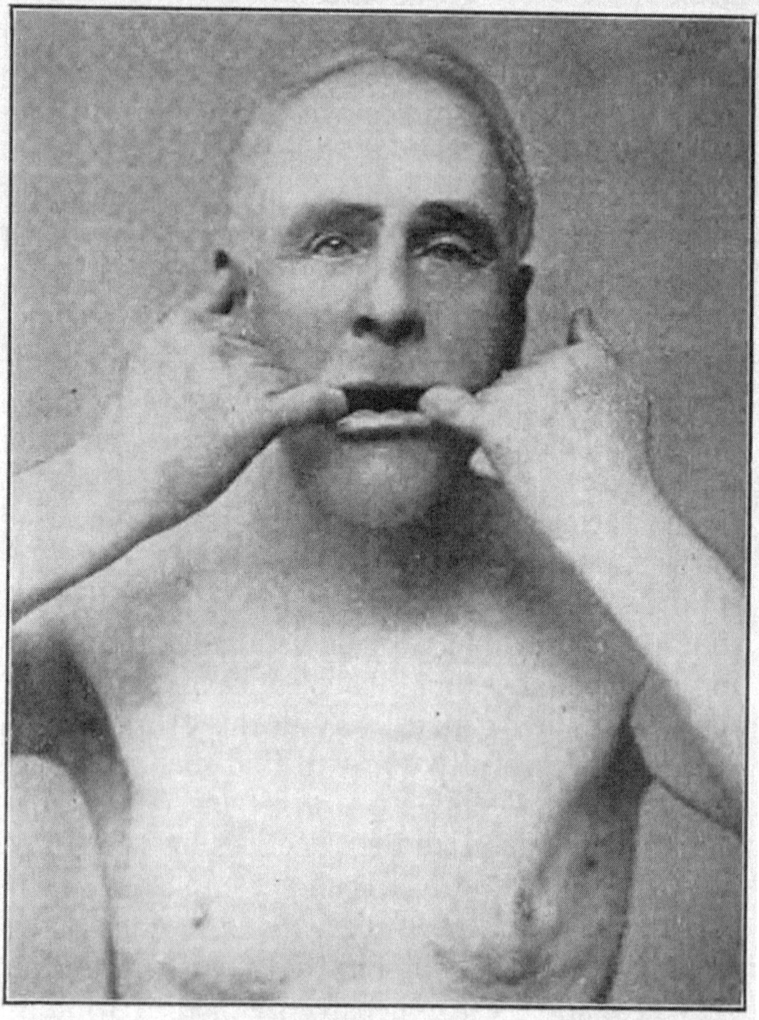

How Drooping of the Mouth is Prevented and Overcome

face with mild soap—the shaving soap used by barbers is best. Dry the face thoroughly, then apply a thin coating of white vaseline; rub off with a dry towel, then a wet one—not dripping wet, but from which the water has been squeezed out so that there will not be a smeary effect. The vaseline will not be absorbed by the skin and but little rubbing is necessary—the dampened towel will aid in cleaning it off, and when "patted" dry with the dry end of the towel the skin will be soft, smooth and not shiny.

Massage of the Face Muscles.—The anatomical illustration on page 251 crudely, but very accurately, shows the muscles of the face which should be exercised; *i. e.* massaged. You will notice the cheeks are supported by eight muscles —four on each side. They are attached to the cheek bones, immediately below the eyes—from that point they descend and become attached to the strong muscle surrounding the mouth and still lower down are again attached to the wide band-like muscles of the jaws. You can contract these supporting cheek muscles at will, this action forming a bunch on the cheek bones, under the eyes. In youth these muscles should support the tissue and skin overlying them, giving to the cheeks the full, smooth appearance characteristic of youth, but as years advance, if they are not exercised, like any other muscle, they will shrink, losing their strength, size and elasticity.

Then as a consequence the skin, not being

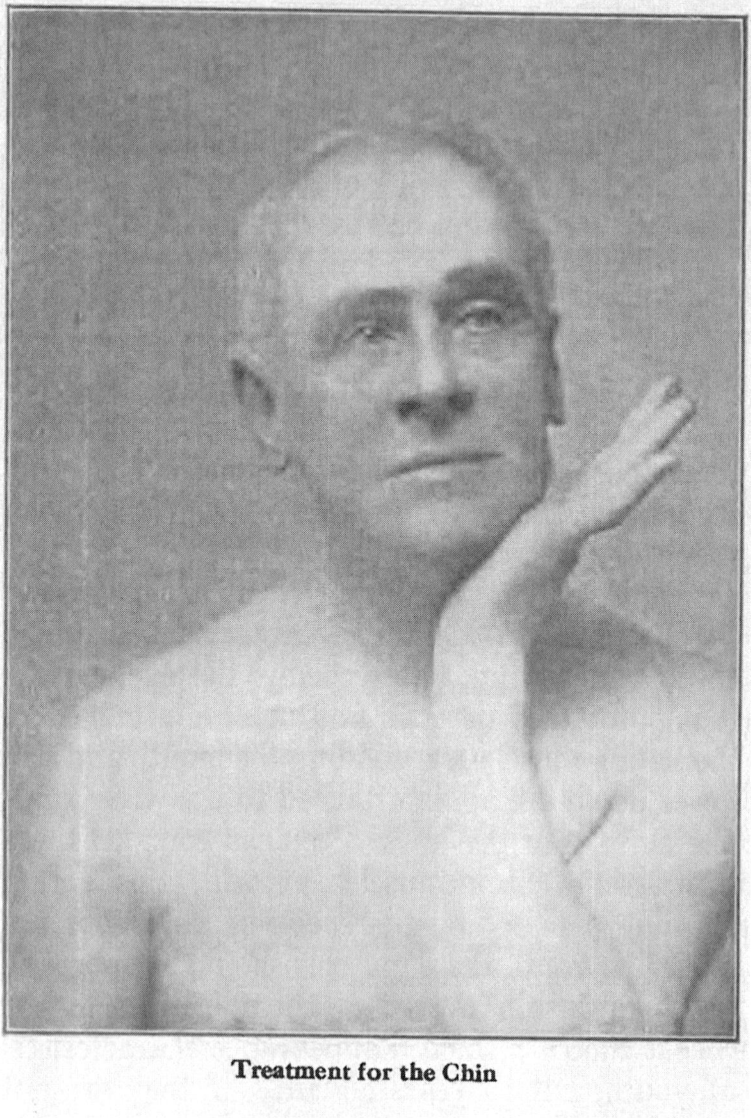

Treatment for the Chin

properly supported, falls into those creases we call wrinkles.

These are the certain indications of physical age, as they tell the tale of the shrunken muscles underlying. For these deep wrinkles, wasted chin and sunken cheeks there can be but one cure, and that is to strengthen and increase the size of those supporting muscles. This can be accomplished by contracting or bunching up the cheek muscles. Then press firmly with the palm of the hand upon the cheek you commence with (see illustration on page 262) and rub those bunched muscles firmly, deliberately and well towards the temples or corners of the eyes.

Ten or fifteen movements will be sufficient to commence with, but gradually increase every morning until you have determined the length of time advisable in your case. After finishing massaging one cheek repeat upon the other; or, if you prefer, practice both at once. This exercise will strengthen the large circular muscle which surrounds the eye and when developed will prevent "sagginess" there. It will also strengthen and develop the cheek muscles; and when this is done the hollows will disappear. In proof of the truth of this statement, I call your attention to the firm condition of the muscles of my cheeks and outline of the jaws.

THE MOUTH.—In the illustrations on pages 251 and 252 you will notice the mouth is encircled by a wide muscular band. As we advance in

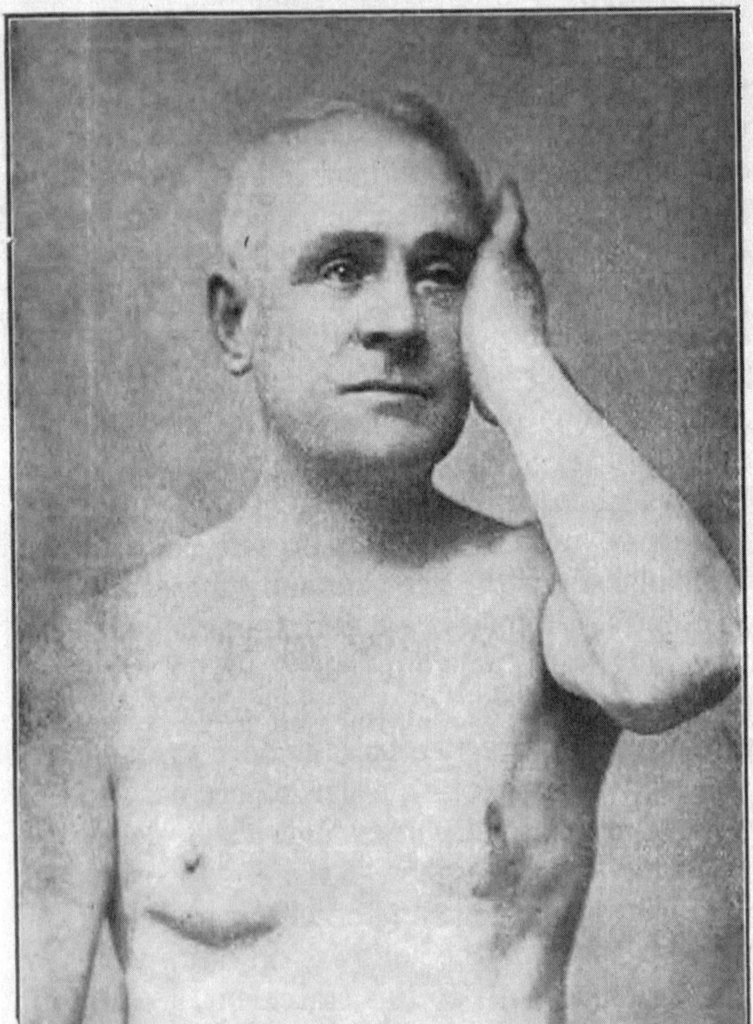

Treating the Temples and the Cheeks

years, if that muscle is not exercised it will atrophy and, becoming weaker, the mouth will sag and droop at the corners—deep lines will then extend from those points downward, the result being the slack mouth of age. You will notice in my full face pictures my mouth does not droop at the corners, but is as firm and muscular as it was when I was fifty years younger. This is due to an exercise I practice for strengthening the "sphincter," or muscle encircling the mouth.

I insert my little fingers in my mouth, as shown in illustration on page 264, then alternately pull and relax. This exercise will speedily strengthen the encircling mouth muscles and the firm mouth which is, or should be, the characteristic of youth will result. This exercise will not stretch and enlarge the mouth, but any droop or sagginess will disappear.

The Chin Muscles.—In connection with the mouth exercise you should endeavor to develop the cushion muscles of the chin. The remedy is persistent firm rubbing of the point of the chin. Also, if lines have commenced to form upon it, dry friction with the palms of the hands and tips of the fingers, as already described, should be practiced. The photograph reproduced on page 266 illustrates my method.

The Temples.—With age the supporting muscles of the temples usually sink and "the sunken temples of age" appear. They should be developed and filled up by exercise; *i. e.*, persist-

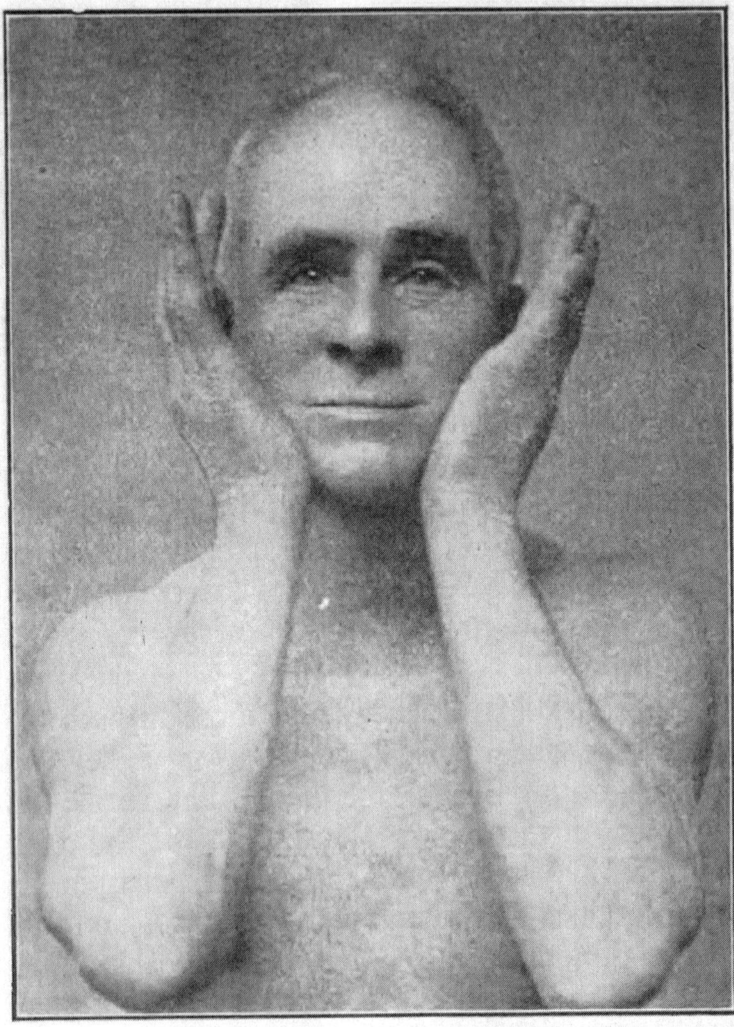

Treatment for the Cheeks and Jaws

ent firm rubbing of these temple muscles, which will remedy this trouble. And frequent friction of the temples well toward the corners of the eyes is advisable. It will produce the smooth temples of youth and also will remove crows' feet. The illustration on page 268 will aid the explanation of the process I advise.

THE JAWS.—Deep, firm rubbing of the muscles of the jaw will develop these muscles. The jaws will then become rounder and a more youthful appearance will result. See illustration on page 270.

I practice all of my exercises, also those for facial rejuvenation, as I lie in bed, in the very early morning, before I "get up," and practice them but once a day. The time I devote to them is about one hour. The mental attitude is a most important factor. For if you have made up your mind to succeed, in "getting young again," you will probably follow my example and therefore make persistent, determined efforts to succeed, then improvement will surely result. While if you think I don't know what I am talking about and have no confidence in my methods, it is not likely that you will. In all exercises, results depend upon yourself.

Massage Exercise for Developing the Cheeks

IN the chapter entitled "Dumb-bell exercises in combinaton with massage of the biceps and triceps," reference is made to the discovery of the athlete, C. A. Sampson, author of "Strength," that the pressure of bands or straps tightly fastened around the arms during exercise speedily increased the size of the muscles. Experimenting, in my efforts to discover the reason why, I found that this pressure during the alternate contraction and relaxations of the muscles, produced a determination of the blood to that point and therefore a distention of the vessels; consequently an enlargement of the structure, just as a sponge will enlarge when its cells are filled with water. Acting upon this idea I substituted the pressure of the palms of the hands for Sampson's bands, and found that in this way the results were the same, and that the muscles of the cheeks could be very speedily enlarged by the following simple exercise, which I practice while lying upon my back. Draw up both corners of the mouth towards the eyes, or in the position of an exaggerated smile. This will bunch up those supporting muscles upon the upper part of the cheek bones immediately below the corners of the eyes. Now drop the chin to its utmost extent. This will place a further tension upon the cheek supporting muscles. In this position, that is, keeping them bunched up, alternately open and close the jaws, at the same time steadily massage, or rub with the palms of the hands. This will infallibly enlarge them, for the logical reasons described and the result will be that the overlying skin and tissue being well supported will give to the cheeks the rounded appearance of earlier years. There will also be an increase in color and a generally improved and more youthful appearance. For the effect of this system upon an old face I again call your attention to the photograph which serves as a frontispiece to this book. At the age of 50 my cheeks were sunken; now, at 72, they are full and round, the result of the persistent practice of the exercise described. It will not produce any lines upon your face, and will certainly develop the supporting muscles of your cheeks, and to the best of my knowledge no other exercise of this nature will.

Massage for the Muscles of the Chin

THE muscles of the chin may be classed as involuntary and can only be developed by massage; but they usually respond more quickly to that process than the muscles that surround the eye.

Rest the chin upon the palms of your hands, press firmly and rub the underlying muscles vigorously; the same method described for the muscles surrounding the eye, but requiring more pressure.

The position of the hands should be continually shifted, for, if continuous pressure is maintained upon any part without relaxation, growth is not so rapid. Change positions, as I have suggested, and if your chin was ever full and round in youth, that condition will, by persistent practice, be regained.

Rapid Development of the Supporting Muscles of the Cheeks

THE instance here illustrated of rapid facial improvement by the persistent and systematic practice of the exercises described, *i. e.*, for the development of the cheek muscles and those of the chin and jaw, is so remarkable that I have obtained the kind permission of the lady who so successfully practiced them to present for the inspection of the readers of this book two photographs. The first was taken July 5, 1909; the second, October 26, 1909, or three months and twenty-one days later. The exercises were commenced and practiced daily and persistently under my directions, and the result has exceeded all expectations of those directly interested in the experiments. This lady was and still is quite slender. Health and digestion were very considerably improved, but not sufficiently to account for the very great change and improvement in her facial appearance. The supporting muscles of the cheeks had greatly atrophied, the cheeks were hollow and the chin emaciated. The face as a consequence presented a thin and haggard appearance. First attempts

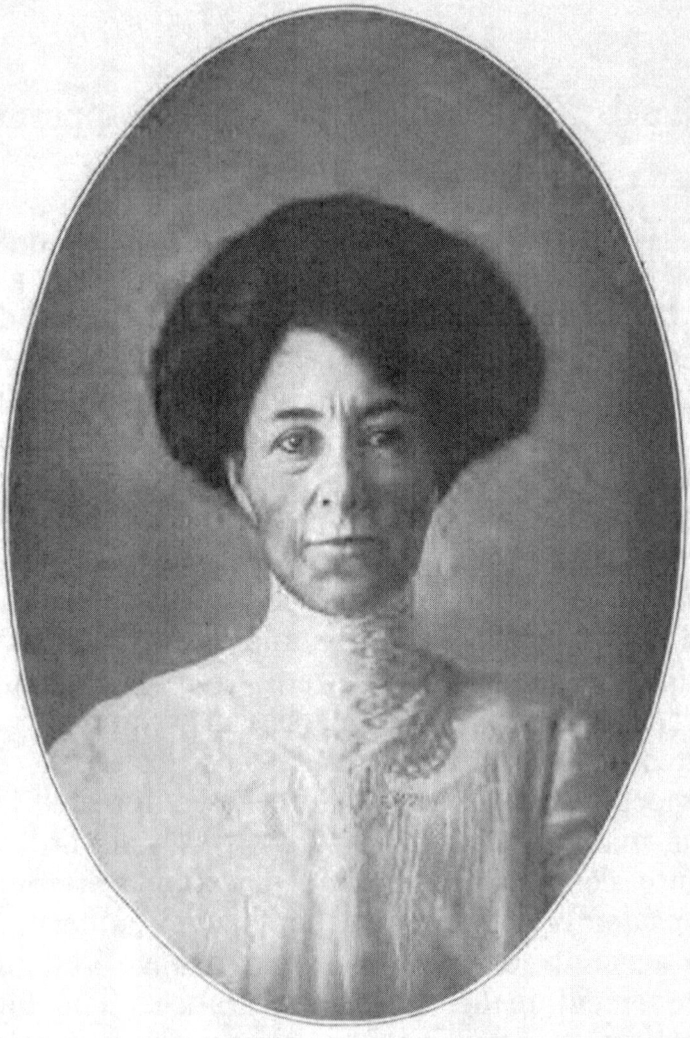

July Fifth, 1909

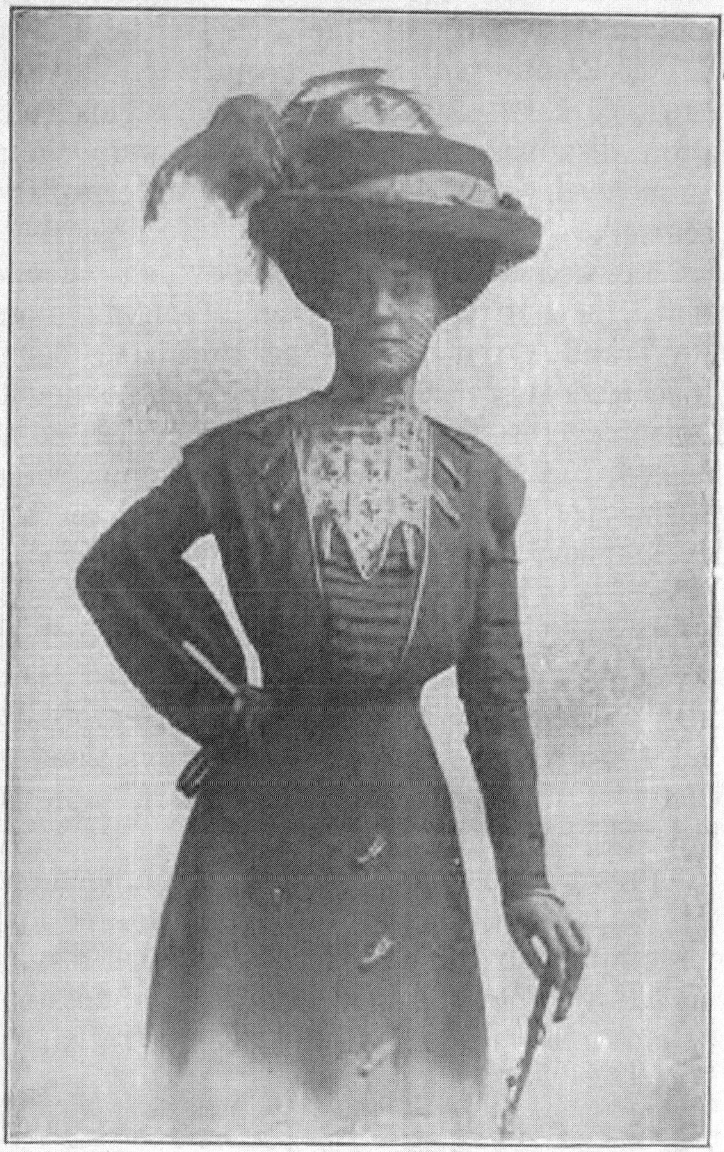

October Twenty-sixth, 1909

at the exercises were not encouraging. The insufficient covering of the bony structure of the cheeks and chin became quite tender, and a rest of three days was allowed. This condition disappearing, the exercises were again commenced, and thereafter no interruption occurred.

A marked improvement was evident in one month, both cheeks and chin becoming more round and symmetrical, the skin also being much improved. The exercises for the development of the throat muscles were then commenced, but improvement at this point, while satisfactory, was not nearly so rapid as the development of the supporting cheek muscles or those of the chin. The reason of this difference in development was, I think, due to the fact of the throat muscles being less atrophied than those of the cheeks and chin. It is also probable that the neck and throat were always slender. Therefore, the apparent difference in rapidity of development.

I present this case for the encouragement of those wishing to experiment in this direction. While no claim is made that such quick results can always be obtained, that it is possible the lady referred to has fully demonstrated.

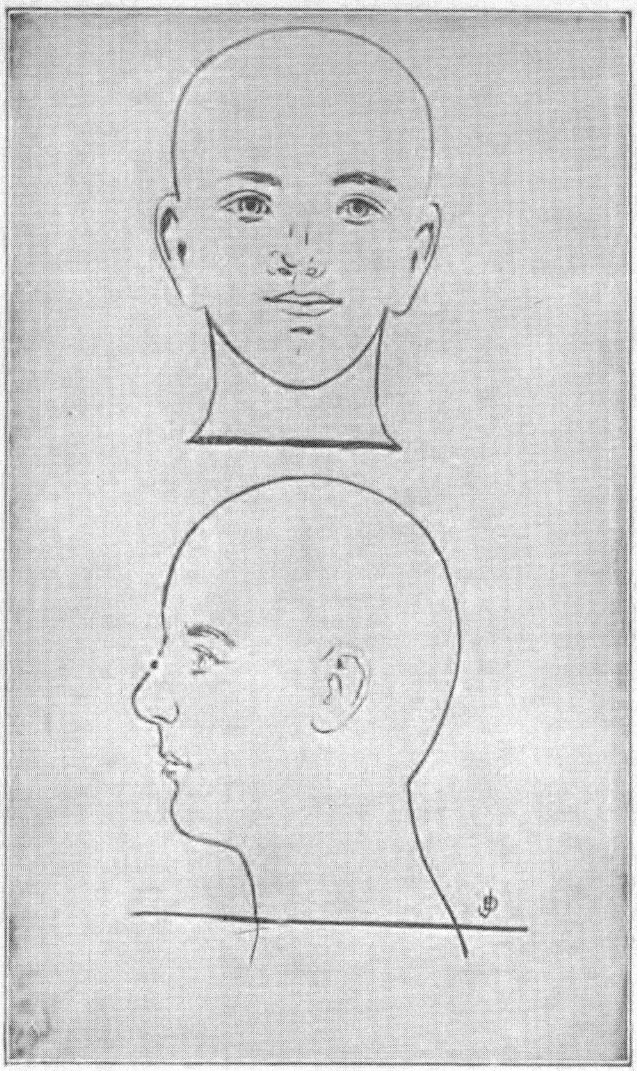

The Smooth Face of a Youth

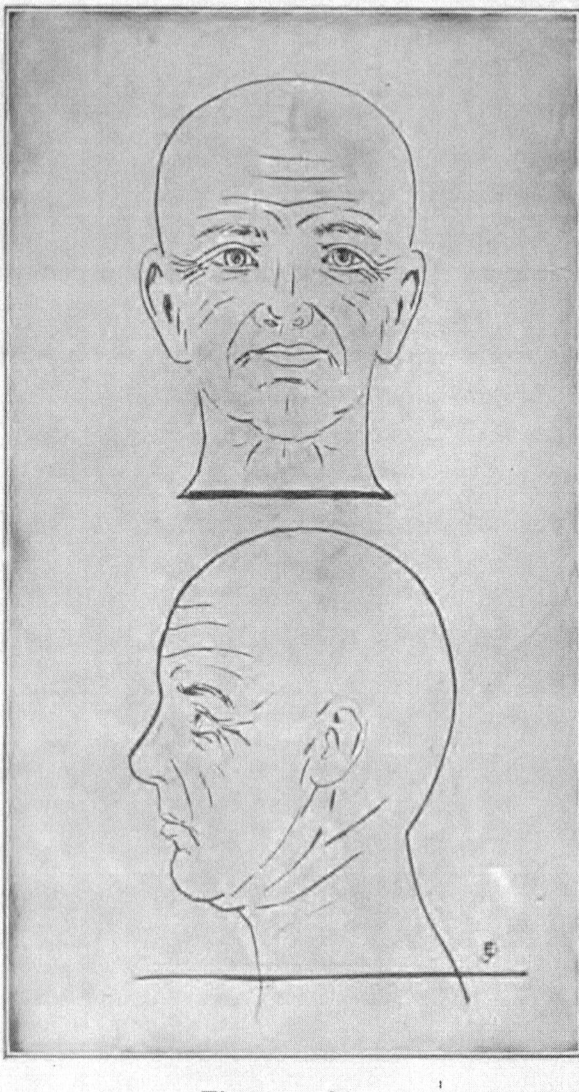

The Lines of Age

The Lines of Age

AS we advance in years certain lines appear upon the face and neck which we associate with age; but these marks of physical deterioration are more often due to neglect than to years. In some women, for instance, they appear at twenty-five; in others, ten years later.

After persistent experiment upon the skin and muscles, for the past seventeen years, I am confident that if the practice of the simple methods described in this book are commenced when the disfiguring lines first appear, it is possible, not alone to efface them, but also to prevent their reappearance until extreme old age.

The preservation of the celebrated beauty of the Sixteenth Century, Ninon de L'Enclos, is a well-known instance of this theory. This woman was remarkable for her wonderful physical preservation. At the age of eighty, creditable authorities state, she retained the great beauty of her girlhood, her face having the freshness of youth, and being as free then from the lines of age as it had been at twenty, her white-powdered hair, then fashionable, but adding to her youthful appearance.

From the data the writer has been able to gather, her smoothness of skin and freedom from wrinkles was due solely to persistent daily friction of the skin of her face, combined with an exercise for the muscles of the neck and throat, very similar to the exercises illustrated and described in this volume. Little was known of the laws of scientific physical culture at that time, but as Madam de L'Enclos retained her elasticity of body and graceful figure to the last, it is evident that some system of exercises was systematically and persistently practiced. In that way alone could her youthful condition have been preserved.

Usually the first marks left by time upon the human features—and they are common to us all—are the wrinkles extending from the nostrils to the corners of the mouth, and beyond. As the years advance these are joined by parallel wrinkles, somewhat shorter, about half an inch distant on the cheek. Still later, another, and even shorter, wrinkle appears at a further distance of less than half an inch; and others are also formed, beginning at the corners of the mouth, and extending downward with a slight inward curve.

Wrinkles on the forehead which parallel the line of the eyebrows, with a slight downward bend at the ends, appear. These are generally from three to five in number, according to one's age. The wrinkles commonly called "crow's feet" spread, fanwise, from the outer corners of the eyes over the temples, and are usually from three to five in number.

The skin below the eyes becomes loose and creased. These creased lines start from the corners of the eyes, slightly curving, and overlapping each other. By this time one or two lines usually appear at the sides of the neck, commencing at a point back of the ears, extending below the jaw, and slanting downward to the throat. Immediately behind the ears, too, the skin becomes slightly loose; two short wrinkles form, and a line appears extending down to, and under, the neck. At the next stage a great number of very short, tiny lines begin to appear all over the face and neck—some parallel, others intersecting. These give to the skin a withered appearance. The freshness of youth has departed. Now, too, the skin under the chin becomes loose; all of the long lines meet and overlay and interweave, and combine with the short ones, just appearing, to form a tangled web of criss-crossings that deepen as the years advance. This is the skein of life. This is the spinning of time. And the pattern is never beautiful!

The only sure method of erasing these lines is by friction, and this is best accomplished with the palms of the hands, as described in the chapter upon the Rejuvenation of the Face and Neck. This treatment, if commenced when the disfiguring lines first appear, and if methodically and daily practiced, in combination with the exercises for the muscles of the face and neck, (described fully in the chapters upon that subject), will surely effect a very marked and satisfactory improvement in the personal appearance.

The Muscles of the Throat

THESE are voluntary muscles and can be exercised at will. They can be increased in size, strength and elasticity. The anatomical illustrations appearing on pages 252 and 292 accurately define the appearance and position of these muscles. Upon them the contour of the throat largely depends. In the illustration on page 252 you will notice a large muscle attached to that projection in the throat known in anatomy as the thyroid bone (more familiarly, Adam's Apple), and from that point ascending to the lower part of the chin, where it is attached. In youth that muscle is usually full, round and elastic, supporting the surrounding tissue and covering skin, filling up the hollows, and giving to the throat the roundness and graceful contour of which the illustration, The Throat of Youth, on the following page is an excellent example.

As years creep on, if that part of the throat is not exercised, this large muscle, and the minor ones surrounding it, following the general law, deteriorate in strength, elasticity and size; the tissue shrinks, and the skin, without its former support, becomes seamed and wrinkled;

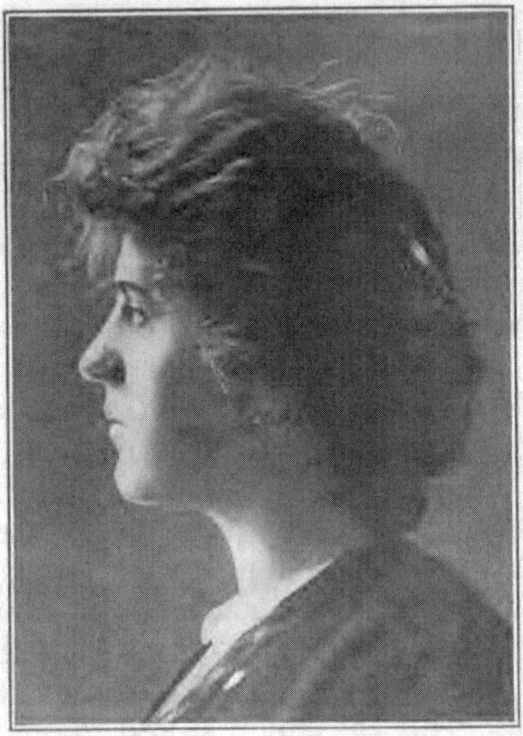

The Throat of Youth

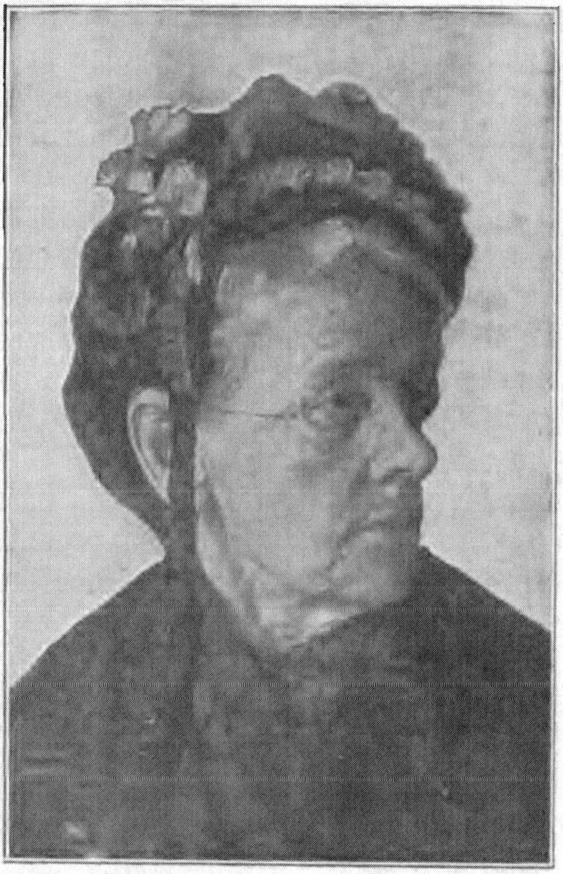

The Throat of Old Age

then, later, falls into loose hanging folds—the throat of old age. (See illustration on preceding page.) If the muscles underlying the loose-hanging skin, as shown in this picture, could be brought back to their former size and condition, it is evident that the contour of the throat would be greatly improved, for it would assume the outline of earlier years. At what age this improvement, by the methods I practice, becomes impossible, I am unable to say. The photograph which faces frontispiece was taken when I was entering my fiftieth year; it shows, under the chin, the loose-hanging skin of age, and that condition remained until I had entered my sixtieth year.

During the period of that ten years, I had industriously and successfully endeavored to improve the rest of my body, but had neglected to exercise the muscles of the throat and face, which consequently presented signs of physical age, in marked contrast to the more youthful appearance of the body and limbs. It being evident that this deterioration was due to the inactivity of these muscles, I devised a system of exercises for their development.

The results of two years' persistent practice in this direction are shown in the profile picture on page 296. The throat muscles have regained their former strength and roundness, and the skin, being well supported, has caused the loose folds, which are shown in the photograph taken twenty-two years ago, to disappear. There is a remarkable improvement over the conditions which then existed. This development of the throat, as well as of the entire neck, has been accomplished with much less exertion, and in less time, than was required to develop the arms and the legs. The most probable reason is, that the throat and face muscles, having never been exercised to any extent, were consequently much atrophied; and this improvement, when they were systematically exercised, was more noticeable. With my personal experience in this direction, I feel warranted in stating that it is possible, and really not difficult, to develop the muscles of the throat and face, by the methods described, after middle age; even after the half-century mark has been passed, wrinkles will disappear, and much of the smoothness of skin characteristic of earlier years may be regained. In short, if you will systematically and persistently practice the methods I have endeavored to make clear, the face and neck will assume a much more youthful appearance.

This will require some exertion upon your part, and some time; but it cannot be accomplished in any other way, all statements of the manufacturer and seller of "skin foods," face ointments, or any rejuvenating preparations, to the contrary. I speak from experience, as I experimented systematically and persistently with various "skin foods" and facial ointments for one year, feeling sure that if I could find any preparation which could be forced through the pores of the skin, and absorbed by the underlying glands, it might be possible to restore to the shrunken muscles of the face and throat the condition of earlier years. The result of that year of experiments was a complete failure, for the reason that the cellular tissue of which these muscles, as well as every other muscle and organ of the body is formed, is the result of the digestion and assimilation of the food we take into our stomachs, the fluids we drink, and the air we breathe. It is impossible to feed or nourish the muscles by any artificial means ever discovered. These so-called "skin foods" or face creams are not absorbed to any appreciable extent, and the improved appearance of the skin after their application is due to the pores of the skin and the myriads of small lines becoming temporarily filled up with the greasy preparation, while the smooth surface is due to the rubbing necessary to apply it. The skin, like any other piece of leather, will polish much better with the palms of the hands, but to avoid chafing should be coated with some smooth face cream or a few drops of olive oil.

There is no royal road to health; it cannot be bought, and if you have ever been endowed with physical beauty, don't waste your time and your money endeavoring to regain it by purchase, for that is not possible.

The rejuvenating methods I have described entail no expense or pain. They are very effective, but their practice rests with you, yourself, and they require both time and patience. If you value your personal appearance sufficiently to work for its improvement systematically and with persistence upon the lines described, my experience is that you will surely succeed. If, however, you conclude, as many will, that it is too much trouble, cultivate a spirit of contentment with your lot, and become resigned to the wrinkles and other indications of physical age, as it is impossible to remove them in any other way than as I have described.

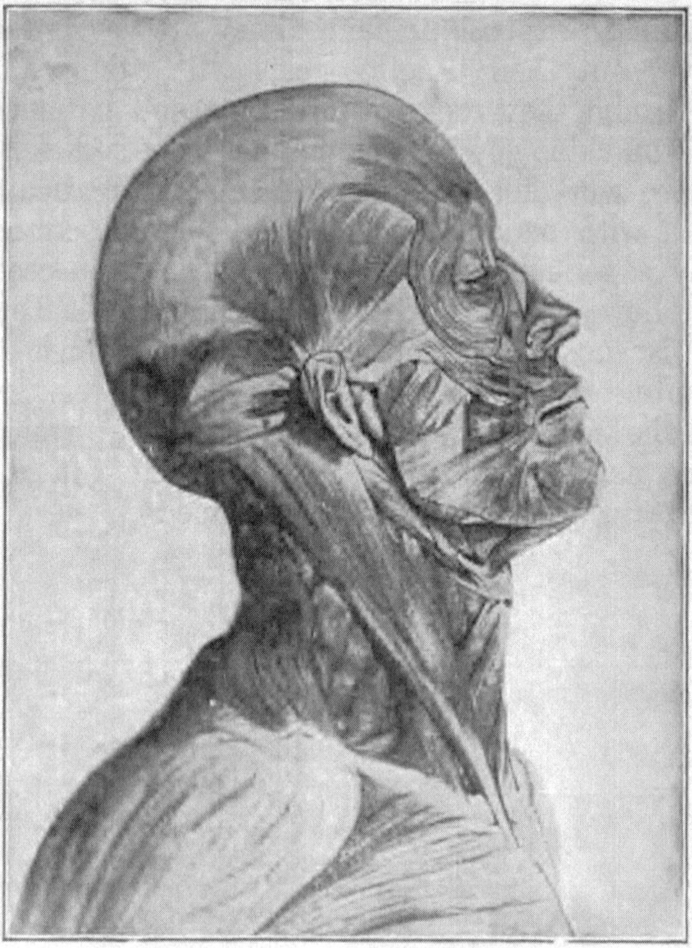

Muscles of the Throat—Head Thrown Back

Developing the Muscles of the Throat—Third Exercise

IT is impossible to present a youthful appearance, if the throat is marred by loose, hanging skin. The face may be free from wrinkles, but if the muscles which support the overlying skin which covers the throat (*i. e.*, immediately below and between the jaws) are shrunken, an appearance of age is inevitable. Therefore, in my efforts at general physical rejuvenation I have endeavored to devise special exercises for the development of the throat and neck muscles. In this direction I have obtained several valuable ideas from a careful study of the methods practiced by Ninon de L'Enclos. The old French pamphlet to which I have previously referred was not altogether clear upon this subject, the description being vague, but evidently the French woman exercised her neck and throat by throwing her head backward, in the position shown in the anatomical plate (page 292). But as the old book stated that she practiced these movements before a mirror, she evidently did so either standing or sitting. Therefore, the head being supported by the

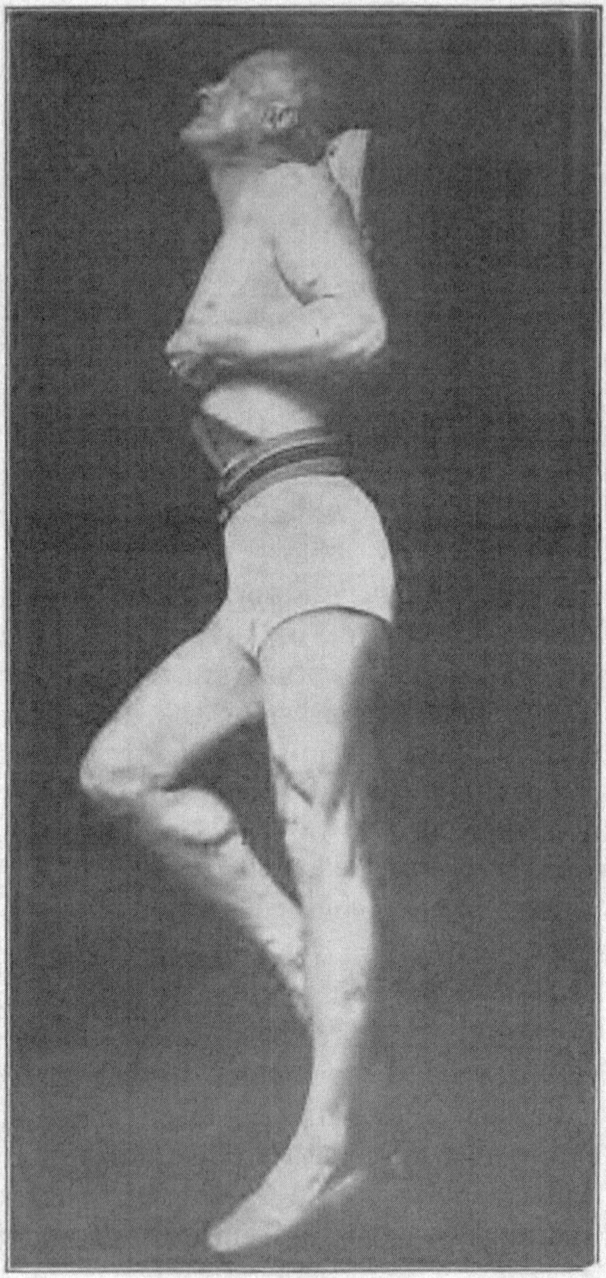

Developing the Muscles of the Throat—Third Exercise

shoulders in both of these positions, the advantage of its weight in the exercises would be lost. I found that by placing a pillow under my shoulders as I lay upon my back, and then throwing the head backward as far as possible (that is, alternately backward and forward), a much greater strain could be placed upon the throat muscles as well as the large ones at the back of the neck. The development in this way would be much more rapid than by the method of the French beauty.

The illustration which accompanies this description will make the position clear. This method of exercising the muscles in question is also less fatiguing than when practiced in an upright position. There is also another advantage. The action of raising the head in the forward motion contracts the abdominal muscles, which relax as the head is dropped back again. This alternate contraction and relaxation is an excellent exercise for these muscles and has a very beneficial effect upon the digestive organs.

Commence slowly, and if any feeling of dizziness results from the unaccustomed activity and position limit your first trials to, say, five movements, but very soon you can attain 100 or more with ease—that is, throwing the head backward as far as possible and then bringing it forward. This is the most effective exercise which can be devised for the purpose described, and if you are really and thoroughly

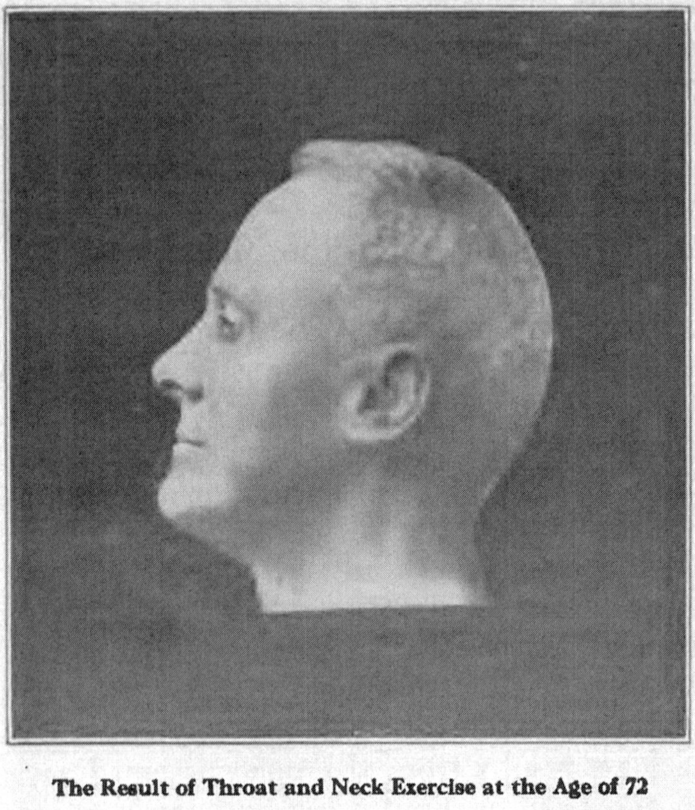

The Result of Throat and Neck Exercise at the Age of 72

in earnest and will faithfully and systematically practice the movements which I have described, you will surely strengthen and round out the neck, and as the muscles of the throat enlarge and the skin overlying them is properly supported, the disfiguring bags will surely disappear.

If the throat is too fat and full—that is, if that *bête noir* of beauty, the double chin, has appeared—this exercise will speedily reduce it. The round, full throat and symmetrical neck of the celebrated French beauty at the age of 70, as shown in her portrait, is a convincing demonstration of the value of these throat and neck exercises. Most probably she never allowed the disfiguring double chin to appear, as she commenced these exercises when physical youth was still hers and continued them throughout her long life. She was able by these means to retain the youthful contour of her beautiful neck and throat to the end.

In my own case I did not commence these special exercises until I was over 50. You will notice that the loose-hanging skin at my throat was very marked at that age (see photograph on first page), while my profile photograph on opposite page, will demonstrate my success at "three score years and ten."

To all women who value their personal appearance I earnestly advise the practice of these three neck and throat exercises. They are the solution of a problem which has puzzled the sex in all ages.

Ninon de L'Enclos

"The Woman Who Never Grew Old"

THE remarkable woman whose portrait appears upon the following page was born in Paris, May 15, 1616; died in Paris, October 17, 1706. She was a convincing and well authenticated example of the truth of the system of facial and physical preservation and rejuvenation as described in this book.

Several of the simple methods of preventing and removing wrinkles, filling up hollow cheeks, rounding the chin and one of the exercises I practice for the development of the muscles of the throat have been evolved from hints obtained from an old French pamphlet published in 1710, the author, Jeanne Sauval, having been the personal and faithful attendant of Ninon de L'Enclos for almost half of a century.

While that old book has no doubt been used as a means of advertising various creams, face lotions and other toilet accessories of doubtful value, and which the great French beauty probably never heard of, yet the exercises therein meagerly and vaguely described, as if they were of no importance, were the real secret of her unprecedented preservation of

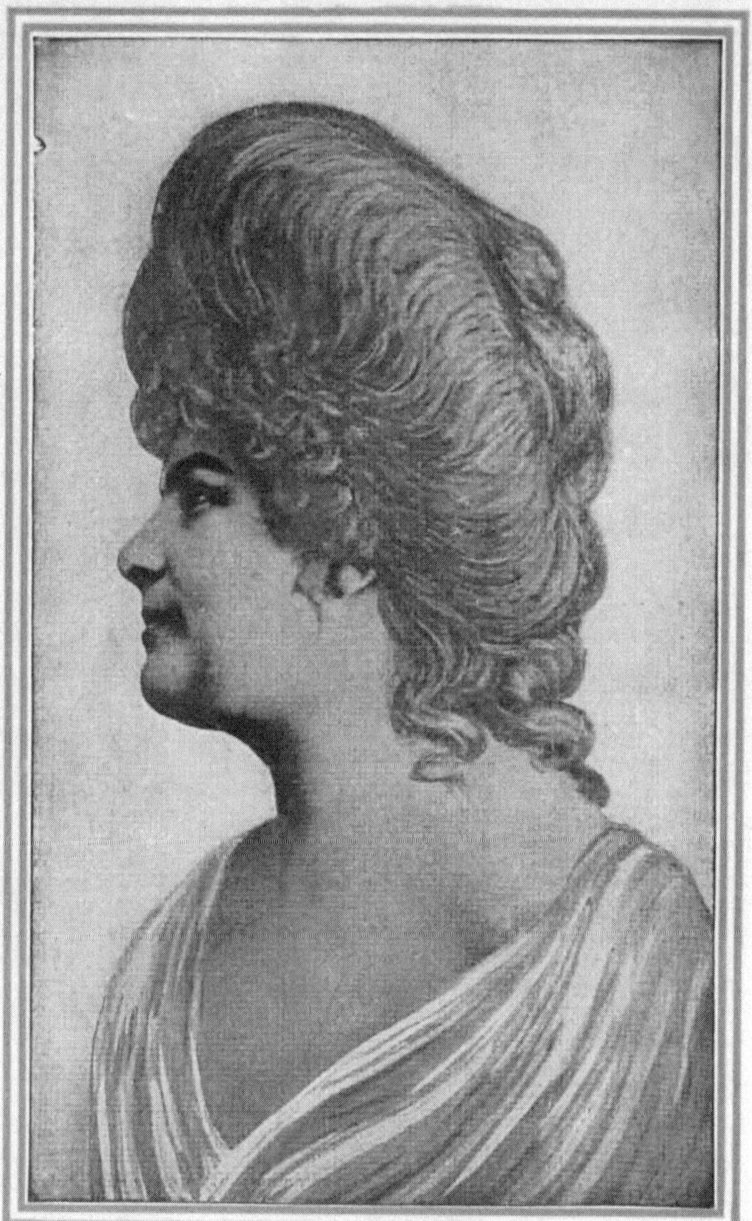

NINON DE L'ENCLOS AT AGE OF SEVENTY
"THE WOMAN WHO NEVER GREW OLD"

apparent youth in advanced years. The metal face mask which her maid states she sometimes wore when sleeping undoubtedly was a very effective aid in the preservation of the smoothness of skin and brilliant complexion described in her memoirs. Yet without the development of the muscles of both face and throat the metal mask alone could not have preserved her youthful appearance at the age of seventy, as shown in her portrait.

This old portrait from which the engraving was taken is still upon exhibition in a celebrated French gallery. It is by Andre Beauchamps, Anno Domini 1686. Therefore the subject of this chapter at the time of that painting had reached her seventieth year. Those interested in the life and personality of Ninon de L'Enclos will find in the American Cyclopedia, Vol. X, under "Len," a long article in reference to her.

For a more extended account of this extraordinary woman see the "Life and Letters of Ninon de L'Enclos," collection and compilation by W. H. Overton, published by the Lion Publishing Co., Chicago, 1903, from which the following extracts are taken:

"Ninon, or Mlle. de L'Enclos, as she was known, was the most remarkable woman that ever lived. For seventy years she held undisputed sway over the hearts of the most distinguished men of France. Louis XIV, when she was 85 years of age, declared that she was the marvel of his reign. Ninon's form was as symmetrical, elegant and yielding as a willow; her complexion of a dazzling white, with sparkling eyes as black as midnight; her teeth like pearls, her mouth mobile, her smile captivating and resistless. Adorable as she was in youth, so she continued to be until her death at the age of 91. An incredible fact, but so well attested by the greatest and most reliable writers who testify to the truth of it, that there is no reason to doubt."

"Ninon attributed it not to any miracle or natural traits, but to her philosophy (that is, her methods of physical and facial preservation), and declared that any one might exhibit the same peculiarities by following the same precepts." (Which statement I fully indorse.)

It is evident that she taught her intimate friends the arts and exercises by which she preserved her marvelous beauty to extreme old age, as the biography further states:

"We have it on the most undoubted testimony of contemporaneous writers who were intimate with him that one of her dearest friends and followers, Saint Evremond, at the age of 89 years, inspired one of the famous beauties of the English court with an ardent attachment."

Of the many portraits painted during the

long life of Ninon de L'Enclos, the picture here presented seems to be the only profile position now extant, and was evidently intended to exhibit the remarkable preservation of her beautiful neck. The full-face portrait which appears as the frontispiece of her memoirs above quoted is now in the gallery of Baron Alfred de Rothschild, painted by Jean Petitot in 1666. She was then about 50. She was evidently much more slender in her youth, or even at the time when the Jean Petitot portrait was painted (at 50), but there is no indication of age in the smooth, round neck and throat, even at three score years and ten.

It is very probable that her luxuriant hair had become gray, as there does not seem to be any effectual method of preventing that mark of age from appearing as we advance in years, but the white powdered hair then fashionable but added to her beauty and youthful appearance.

This picture, with the statements given, is presented as indisputable evidence that if the human body is through life kept free from wornout tissue, dead cells or other clogging matter it will not exhibit what we know as "the signs of age"' to a period long past that which we now think to be the physical limit of the appearance of youth.

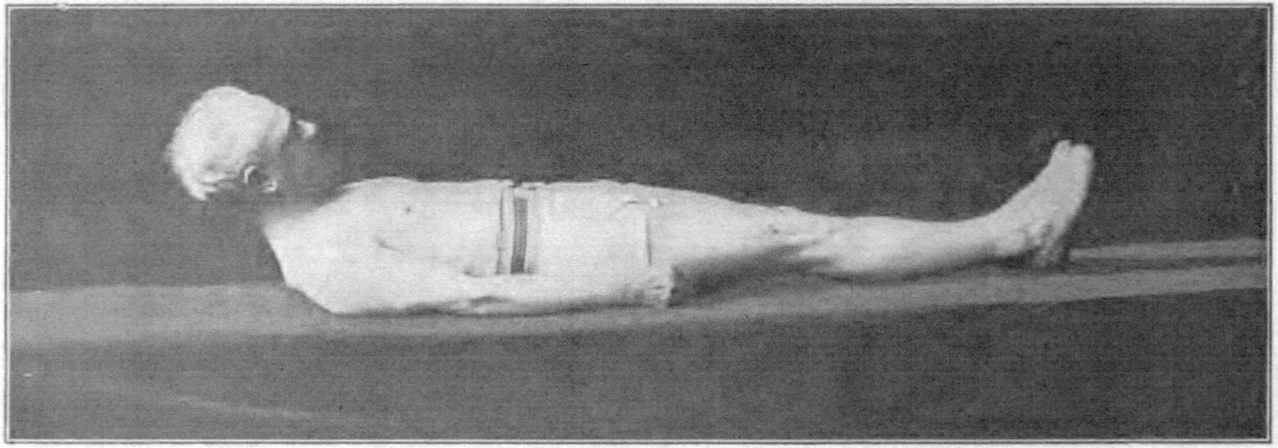

Muscles of the Back of the Neck and Abdominal Muscles

Muscles of the Back of the Neck and the Abdominal Muscles

LYING upon the back, as shown in the illustration, when you raise your head you will find that a tension is placed upon all of the muscles of the neck, but particularly those at the back of the neck. The large, flat muscles which brace up the abdomen are also brought into action.

To exercise and strengthen both of these very important sets of muscles, lie upon your baek and alternately raise and lower your head. Five movements will be sufficient to commence with, but as your strength increases ten times that number will not tire you and can do no harm.

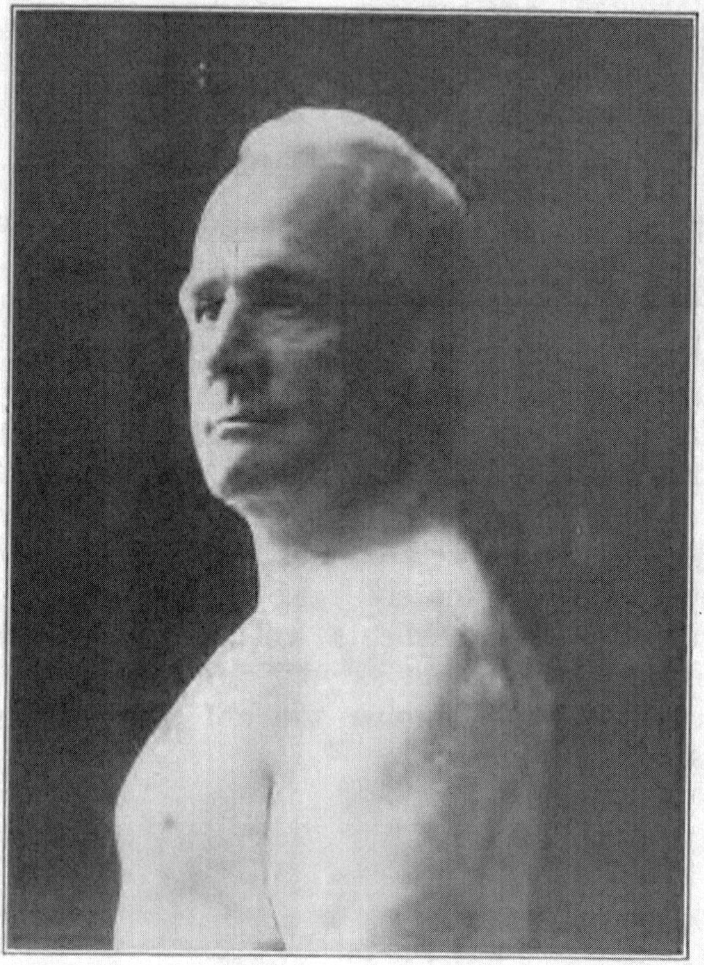

Development of Neck Muscles
Sanford Bennett at Age 67

The Skin

THE skin forms a protective covering, a close-fitting garment, for the whole body. It is of unequal thickness; over those parts which are exposed to pressure and friction it is thick and tough, but in the case of other parts liable to variations in size it is especially elastic. But in every place it is adapted to the purpose of protection.

It is both a secreting and an excreting organ, and upon its proper action our health, our very lives, depend. If its millions of glands and pores become obstructed it is impossible for one to be healthy. On the other hand, when these openings—the safety valves of the body—are free and clear, the impurities of the body are readily thrown off, the circulation is improved, an equilibrium is established in the eliminating process between the skin and the internal organs, digestion is easier, intestinal and urinary secretions become more regular, and an improvement in the nervous condition results. My own experience has been that daily friction of the skin with goat-hair mittens and a goat-hair friction belt will materially relieve insomnia. These friction exercises should be followed by a tepid bath. The moral of it all is: Keep the skin clean by friction and bathing.

The skin is composed of three layers. Overlying the true skin is the cuticle, or scarf skin, and although we commonly call this the *skin*, it is really only a protecting layer over the true skin. It has no blood vessels, so it never bleeds; and, as it contains no nerves, it feels no pain. The microscope shows that it is composed entirely of minute flat scales which overlap each other very much like the shingles of a roof. These scales are formed by the true skin beneath, and are constantly thrown off from the body. Ordinarily this is imperceptible; but sometimes the scales accumulate into masses, when it is called scurf. Or, if the accumulation is upon the scalp, it is known as dandruff.

Upon the condition of the scarf skin the complexion largely depends. If it is rough, a good complexion is impossible. Temporary improvement can be obtained by use of the remedies dear to the feminine mind—"skin foods," face creams and face powders. But all of these applications have the same result: they simply fill up the minute lines, and temporarily smooth the rough surface. But when this coating is washed off, the skin will resume its former condition.

It is not usually claimed for face powders that they will afford more than a temporary improvement, but the manufacturers and venders of so-called "skin foods" positively assert that their preparations feed and nourish the skin, and build up the underlying muscles, and that the benefit derived from their use is therefore permanent. If lanoline, paraffine, white wax and spermacetti, the basis of all these preparations, could be forced into the true skin and the muscles, and could there be converted into living cellular tissue, of which all parts of the body (the skin included) are composed, this claim might have some foundation of truth. But as these cells can only come into life by the process of digestion and assimilation, the fallacy of the above claim is apparent. You certainly cannot form or "build up" living tissue from dead matter. The term "skin food" is a very attractive title for these greasy, waxy preparations, but neither the skin nor the muscles can feed on that kind of food. By friction some very slight superficial absorption of the higher grades of oil is possible; but even this does not become living tissue. As this absorption is limited to only the very highest grades of oil, it is manifestly impossible for the skin to take up paraffine, white wax, or any of the other coarse concomitants of "skin foods."

Their immediate effect, as before stated, is to coat the surface of the skin, which, after their use, assumes a smoother appearance. But this is temporary, and there can be no growth or improvement of the underlying muscles by such applications. The objection to these greasy ointments is that they clog up and obstruct the myriads of underlying pores and glands. If you would have a healthy skin, these outlets for the impurities of the system must be kept clean and clear. Otherwise the skin cannot be healthy.

The secret of a fresh, healthy skin is friction and cleanliness. Upon the body use the goat-hair friction mittens and the friction belt of the same material. It is advisable that these friction exercises be practiced daily—after the other exercises described in this book—and followed by a tepid bath.

For the face and neck, friction with the palms of the hands is an effective method of removing wrinkles, as they can be rubbed out, and the skin can be polished, as elsewhere stated, just like any other piece of leather. For the ablutions of the face and neck use tepid water softened with borax.

In a very short time after commencing these friction exercises for the body, you will find that the nervous system is quieter and that both the digestion and the circulation are improved. And what will prove of special interest to ladies is that the friction exercises for the face and neck will surely result in a marked improvement.

I have demonstrated upon my own face and neck that by this method wrinkles can be removed even in advanced age, and I am positive that if this friction exercise is commenced when the lines first appear and is persistently practiced, they will be eradicated and will not again appear until extreme old age. This is the method that was practiced by Ninon de L'Enclos, the celebrated French beauty of the seventeenth century, and it is the only successful method for removing wrinkles and retaining the smooth skin characteristic of youth. For the details of the rejuvenation of the face and neck, see the chapter under that title.

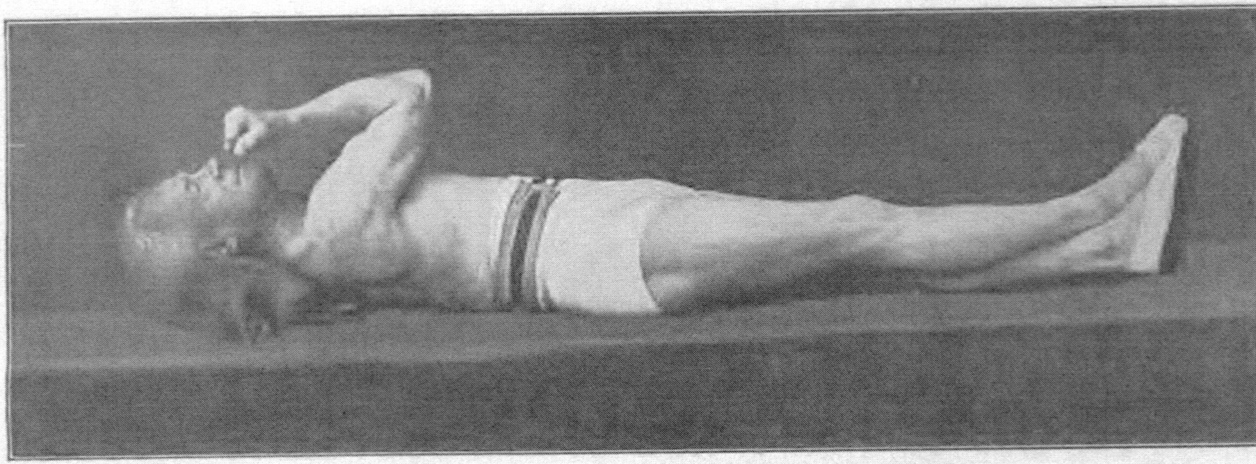

Exercising the Muscles Which Cover the Shoulder Blades

Exercising the Muscles Which Cover the Shoulder Blades

LYING upon your back, as shown in the opposite illustration, strike with your elbow across the chest. This movement will bring into action and develop the muscles covering the shoulder blades. Five movements for each arm will be sufficient to commence with. This exercise is valuable where there are any indications of acid rheumatism in the muscles described. I speak from personal experience.

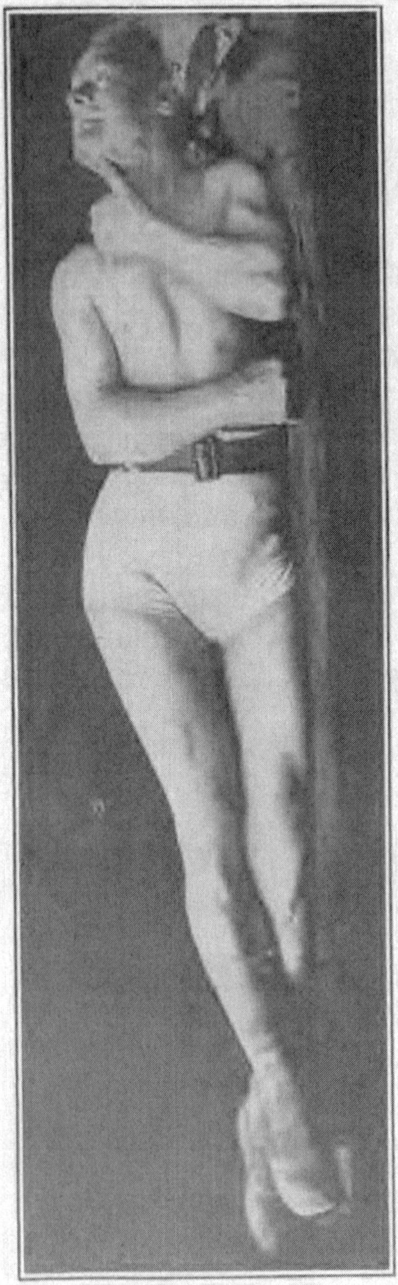

Developing the Throat Muscles

Exercise for the Development of the Throat Muscles

First Exercise

LYING upon your side, place your thumb on the throat immediately under the chin, or at about the center of the large muscle which extends from the Adam's Apple to the chin (see anatomical plate on page 292). If you lie upon your right side, use the right thumb; if upon the left, use the left thumb. Throw the head back to the position shown in the illustration on the opposite page.

Then bring the head forward (chin to the chest) which will relax the tension. Keep up the pressure of the thumb while alternating, contracting and relaxing the muscles by the movements described. This movement will tense the muscles of the throat, which the exercise is intended to develop, the firm, upward pressure of the thumb adding to that tension.

Commence with ten movements each morning, increasing gradually, as your physical condition will warrant, to fifty.

This exercise should be practiced while recumbent, both upon the right and left sides. If practiced faithfully and systematically a marked improvement of the contour of the throat will surely result.

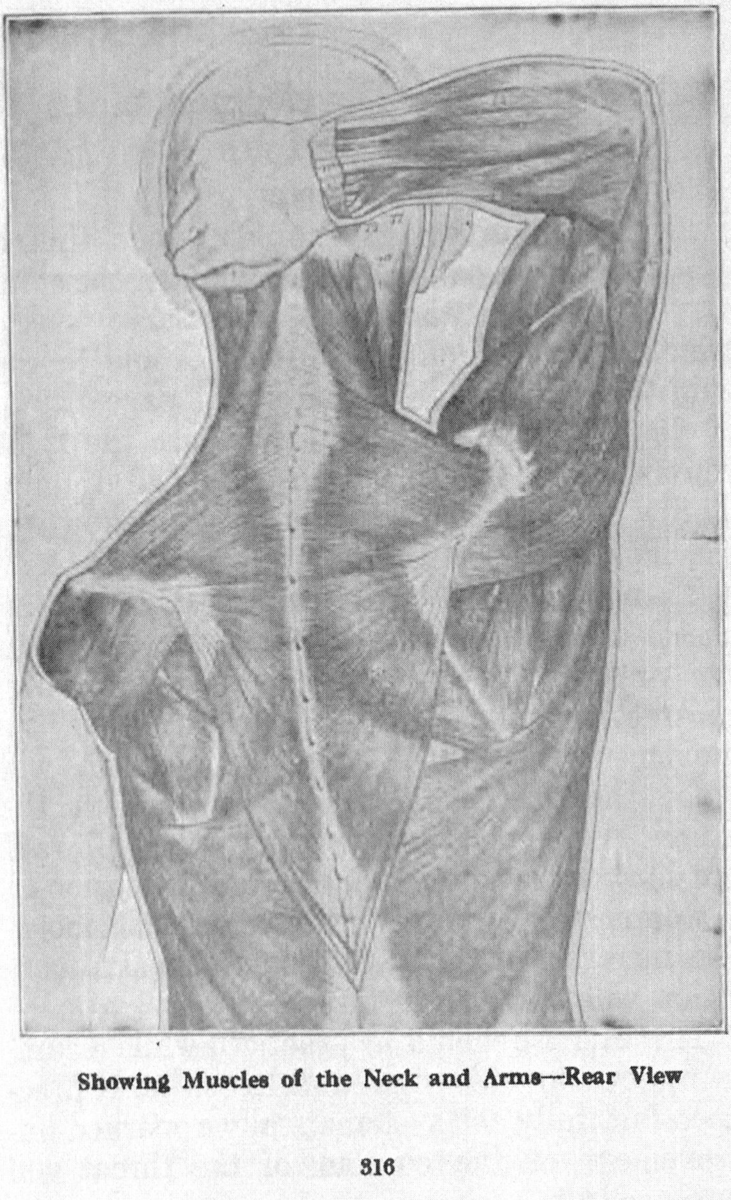

Showing Muscles of the Neck and Arms—Rear View

The Neck

THE principal supports of the neck are two large muscles attached to the base of the skull, and from thence descending to the shoulders; they form the back of the neck. The sides are braced by another pair of large muscles which are attached to the skull immediately behind the ears, and which descend to the collar bone. These large muscles are braced by minor ones, but upon these main supports the contour and strength of the neck largely depend. If they are poorly developed the back and sides of the neck will appear weak and unsymmetrical; the skin-covering, lacking the proper support, will soon fall into unsightly creases; and in this condition there is an appearance of age which the time of life may not warrant.

Persistent rubbing of the back and sides of the neck with the palm of the hand will, to a considerable extent, efface these wrinkles; but this is a superficial treatment and its effect is but temporary; as, if the underlying muscles are shrunken and weak, the skin—being poorly supported—will surely become loose and flabby, and the creases will deepen.

The remedies dear to the feminine mind for

this condition are so-called "skin foods" and other greasy preparations of like nature. But as it is impossible to form muscular tissue by their use, the fallacy of the process is evident. The skin will certainly be improved by the friction necessary to apply the preparations, but aside from this the treatment is of no avail.

It is evident that if the muscles described were developed and restored to the condition of earlier years, the skin, being then properly supported, would regain its smooth surface. This can be accomplished by practicing the several exercises for both neck and throat which are described.

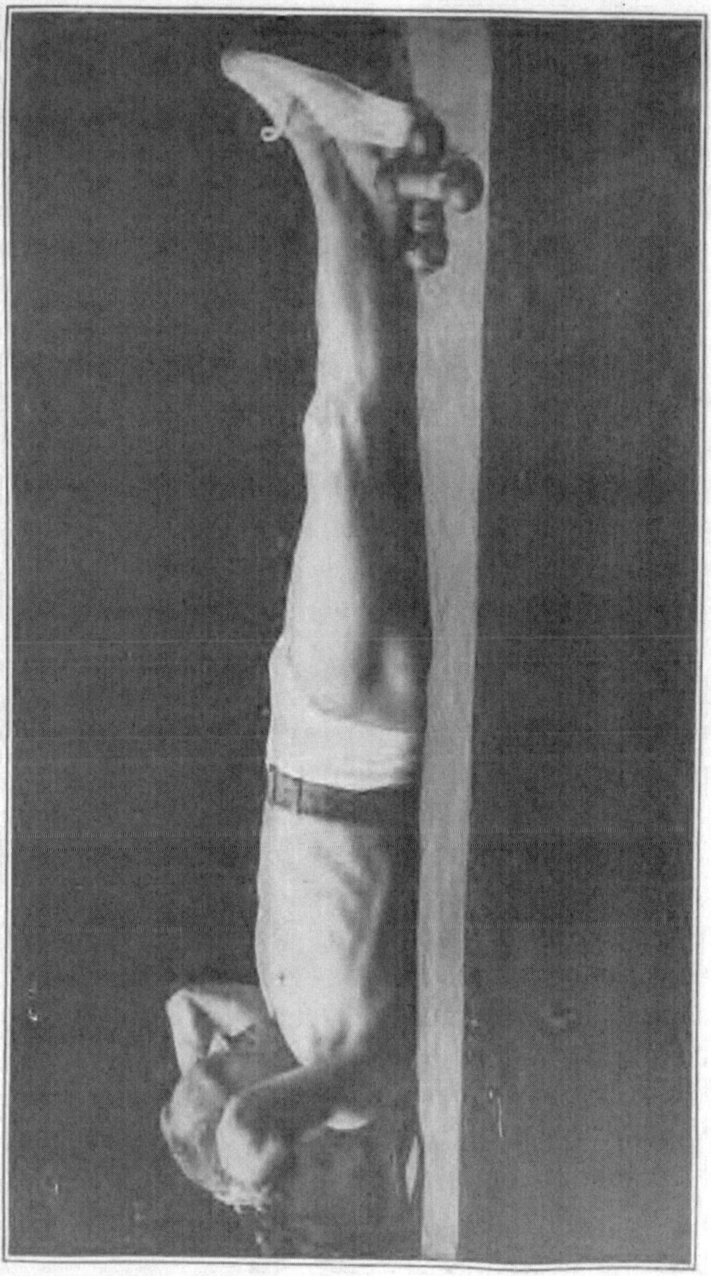

Developing the Muscles of the Neck

Exercise for Developing and Strengthening the Neck

CLASP the hands firmly back of the head, as shown in the illustration on preceding page. Raise the head clear of the pillow; then press it backward, exerting at the same time a strong forward, or resistance, pressure with the arms. Commence with not more than five movements; that is, alternately raising and lowering the head, at the same time keeping up the full strain of the arms. At the end of a week increase one or two movements, as your condition may warrant. My own limit is now twenty-five, which I find ample. By an excess of this exercise, I increased my neck measurement from fourteen to sixteen inches; which, being out of proportion to my height (see illustration on page 306), I totally discontinued for about six months, the same measurement reducing to fifteen and one-quarter inches; at which it remains.

The muscles called into action, and specially developed by this exercise, are shown in the illustration on page 292.

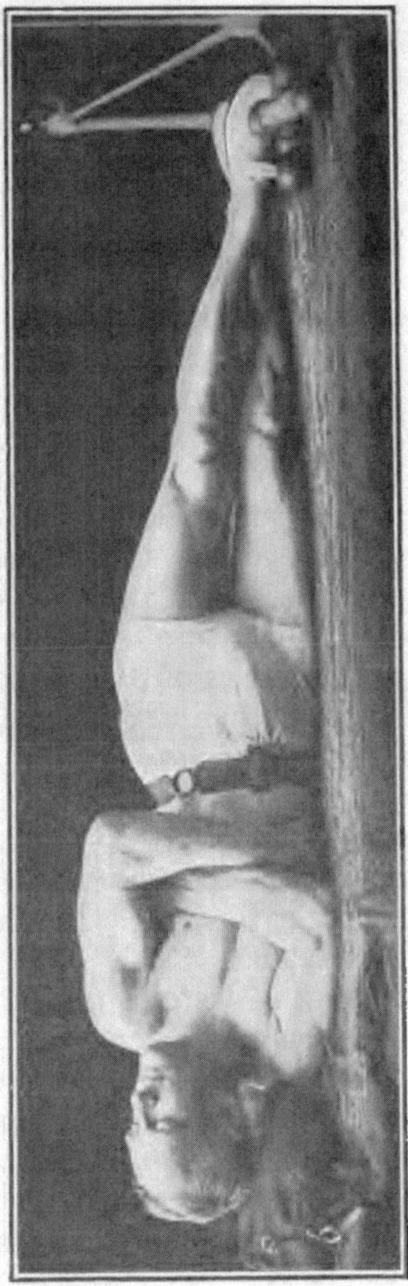

Developing the Muscles of the Neck

Developing the Sides of the Neck

LYING upon your side, as shown in illustration on preceding page, turn the chin as far as possible towards the upper shoulder. (This movement will contract the muscles upon the side of the neck, and will also bring into action those muscles of the throat immediately under the chin.) When the head drops back to its original position the muscles will relax. Their alternate contraction and relaxation constitute an exercise which will develop the muscles of the sides of the neck, and will also strengthen and improve the contour of the throat muscles.

Commence the exercise with five movements, and increase to fifty or more, as your physical condition improves. Both sides of the neck must be exercised, for otherwise the development will be unequal.

The effect of this exercise upon the neck is shown in the illustration on page 306. The deep lines which once crossed and re-crossed the back of my neck have wholly disappeared, and my appearance at this point is that of a man of half my years.

Ladies who may contemplate practicing this

exercise need not fear the appearance of undue muscularity which this picture exhibits. The effect of exercise upon the muscles of women is not the same as upon the muscles of men. The knotted and rugged appearance of the muscles of the trained male athlete never appear in women, although similarly trained. Their muscles always remain soft, elastic and more graceful in their roundness than those of men.

The exercise here described will improve and beautify the neck at a time when, in middle life, it is usually very scrawny.

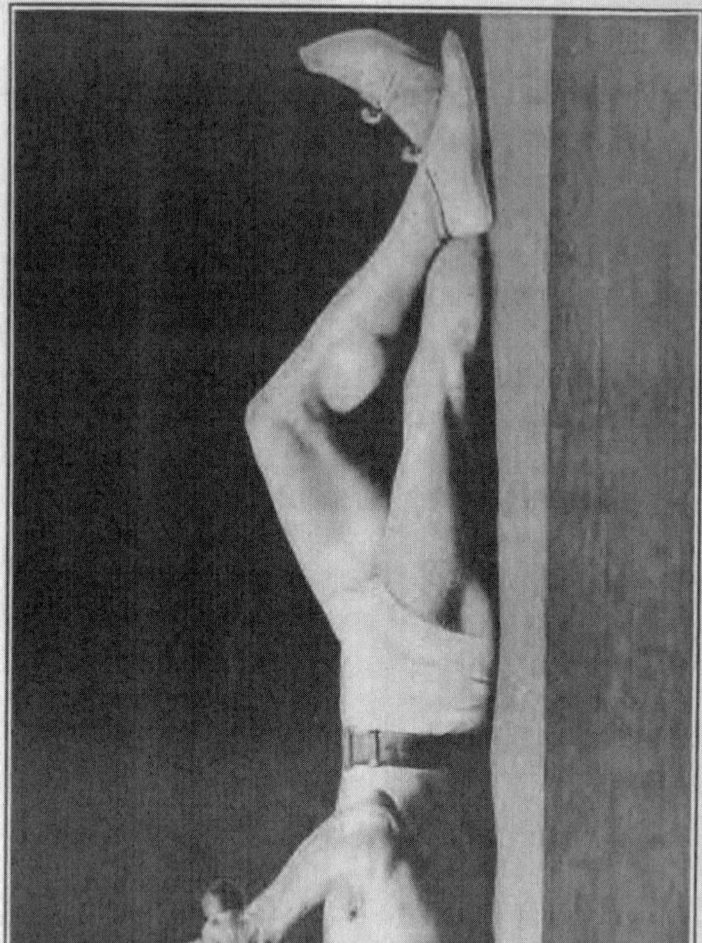

Developing the Arms by Dumb-Bell Exercise

Dumb-Bell Exercise for Two Hands

I STRONGLY advocate the use of light dumb-bells. The pair I use weigh four pounds, but half that weight, in most cases, will be sufficient. I have experimented, as I lay in bed, with all sizes up to forty pounds, but I have found moderately quick action with weights of from two to four pounds the most effective. There is always a danger of over exercise with the heavy dumb-bells; the continuous strain may affect the heart, and certainly has a tendency to bring on that condition known in athletics as being "muscle bound."

The light weights with rapid action, in the position shown by the illustration upon the opposite page, will give an elasticity and general quickness of motion which cannot be obtained with the heavy dumb-bells.

Commence with ten strokes; increase, as your condition will warrant, to fifty or more. It is a safe and effective exercise. After this striking exercise is completed, extend your arms to their full length at right angles with the sides, and alternately turn, or twist, your wrists back and forth, so that the arms will partially revolve in their shoulder sockets. If there is any tendency to rheumatic pains at this point, where deposits of uric acid frequently occur, this movement will be found to be beneficial, as it will dislodge such deposits.

Commence with five movements and gradually increase to twenty-five, which at all stages will be sufficient.

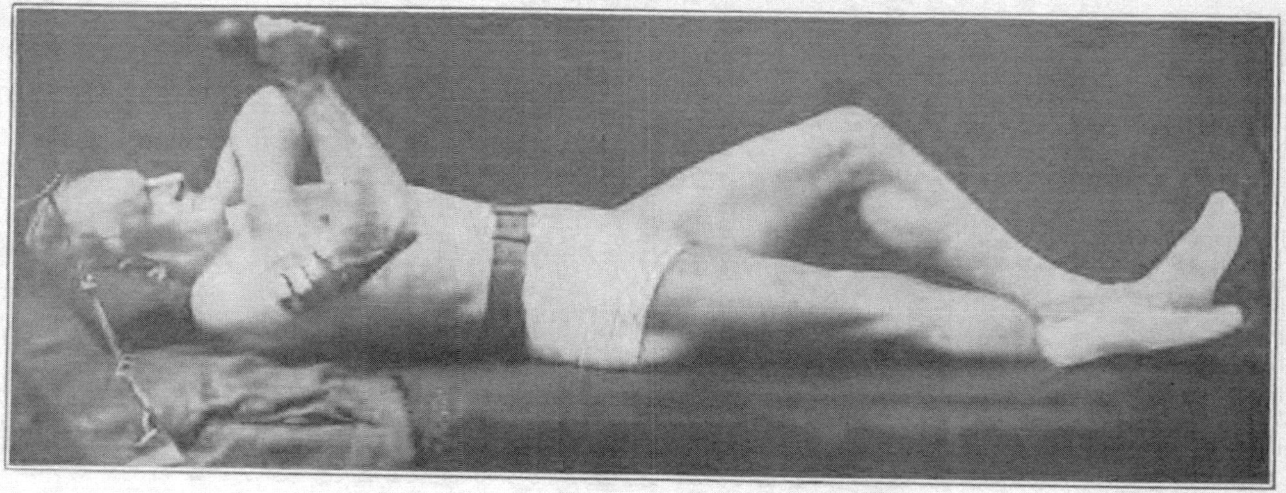

Developing the Arms by Dumb-Bell Exercise and Massage

Dumb-Bell Exercise

In Combination with Massage of the Biceps and Triceps Muscles

DEVELOPMENT of the arms, by this method of exercise, is very much more rapid than by boxing, or any gymnasium exercise practiced with the usual mechanical appliances.

To the celebrated athlete, C. A. Sampson, one of the world's strong men and the rival of Sandow, seems due the credit of discovering that massage of the muscles during exercise greatly aids their development. The method employed by him was the application of strong elastic bands or straps, which he fastened tightly around his arms during his dumb-bell exercise. The alternate pressure and relaxation of the bands or straps, as the muscles were contracted or relaxed, made a very effective massage. He attributed his marvelous strength to this practice.

After studying his method, and the very logical reasons he advances in his book, "Strength," I procured the elastic straps described and practiced according to his directions. The improvement that resulted was soon apparent, and it was evident that the system would effect all that its author claimed for it, but the inconvenience of the device was such that I abandoned it. I substituted the exercise shown on page 327, using, instead of the elastic straps or bands, simply the pressure of the hands clasped firmly over the upper arm, which I massage while I am using the dumb-bell.

Development of the biceps and triceps muscles will be found to be very rapid by this system.

Commence practice with not more than ten movements; then increase gradually to fifty for each arm; this, with daily practice, should be sufficient to keep the arms strong and flexible. Weight of dumb-bells two to four pounds, in accordance with your strength. In traveling or under circumstances where the dumb-bells cannot easily be procured, this exercise can be performed very effectively without them.

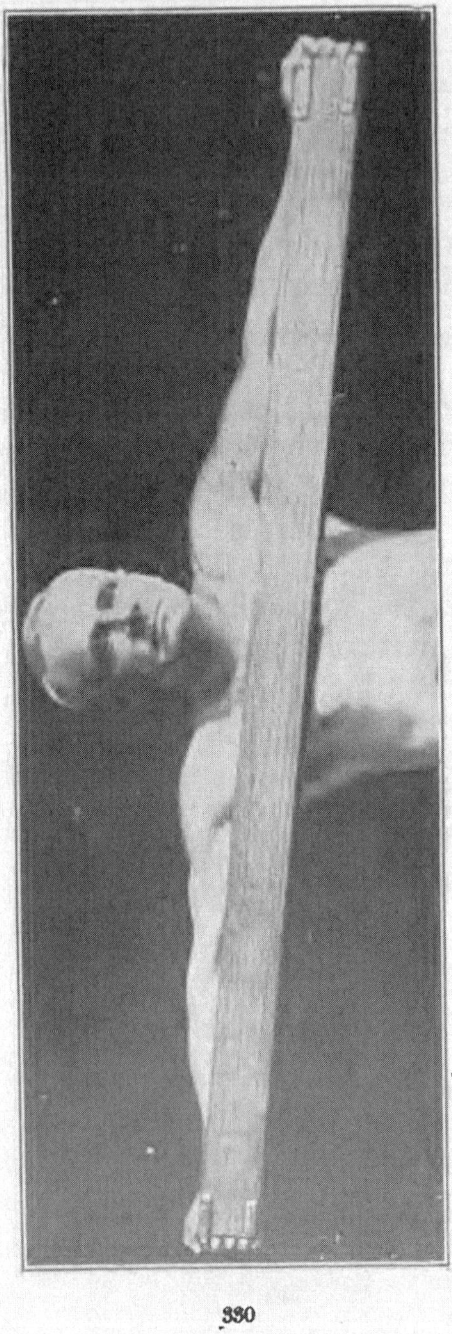

Using the Stretching Board

Stretching-Board Device for Broadening the Shoulders

THIS exercise is only intended for exceptional cases; *i. e.*, those whose shoulders are abnormally narrow. The shoulder stretching board was originally devised for a young man who was notably deficient in this respect. His success in its use decided me to describe and illustrate it as in the foregoing pages. The board is easy to make, inexpensive and very effective for the purpose described.

In most gymnasiums there is an excellent exercise practiced to broaden the shoulders by the means of lateral tension. Standing between two upright parallel bars, the student grasps them with both hands, his arms outstretched at right angles to the body. The exercise consists in pulling alternately with either hand, first right, then left. This action exercises or stretches laterally the muscles of the shoulders, and, if regularly and persistently practiced, improvement is certain.

At the commencement of my efforts to devise simple methods in exercising in bed, as a substitute for the regular gymnasium exercise, I unsuccessfully experimented with rings, bars and ropes, which I attached to the sides of the bed, endeavoring to effect lateral tension of the shoulder muscles by such means. I found that, in addition to the inconvenience of the fixtures, the body was unpleasantly shifted from side to side by the force of the pull; while the desired result, directly contrary to that, was an alternate tension and relaxation of the shoulder muscles, without any change in the position of the body.

Finally I tried a board, as long as the spread of my outstretched arms and three inches in width. This I grasped at the ends, the pull of the opposing hands giving the lateral tension of the shoulder muscles without disturbing the position of the body. I found this stretching board very effective, and the only improvement I have ever made upon it is to attach strong iron handles to the ends, that the hands may have a firmer and more convenient hold.

The Exercise Is This

Lying upon your back, with the board resting diagonally across the chest, the hands grasping the ends or handles, as in the illustration on page 230, pull with your full force upward as far as possible, that the muscles under the arms and extending along the upper ribs may receive the strain; resist with a downward pull of equal force; next reverse the pull, that each side may be exercised.

Second Movement

With the board lying at right angles across the chest, pull with both hands at once, keeping up the strain for two or three seconds; then relax. Commence with five movements for each exercise; that is, alternately tensing and relaxing the muscles, as described; increase to fifteen movements, as your physical condition may warrant.

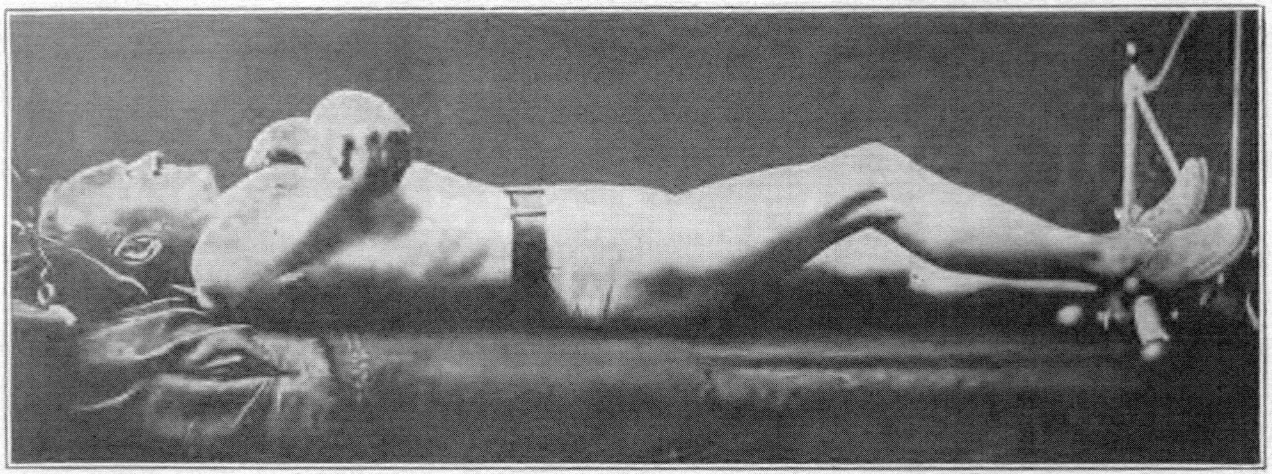

Broadening the Shoulders

Exercise for Broadening the Shoulders

LYING upon your back, grasp the left elbow with the right hand, and the right elbow with the left hand. (As pressure is exerted, you will feel an outward or lateral strain upon both shoulders.) The upper arms, under this cross pull, act as levers forcing them apart; the pressure from the right hand upon the left elbow acts upon the shoulder muscles of the left side, while a corresponding effect takes place upon the opposite shoulder. In this position, practice that motion familiarly known as shrugging the shoulders; the lateral strain and tensed condition of the muscles, combined with the up and down movement of the shoulders, is a most effective method of developing that part of the body.

Commence with five movements, increasing daily, as your strength and physical condition will warrant, until you have reached twenty-five with ease, and without any feeling of soreness. This is a very good and effective exercise, and will surely have the desired result if persistently practiced. (See illustration on page 334.)

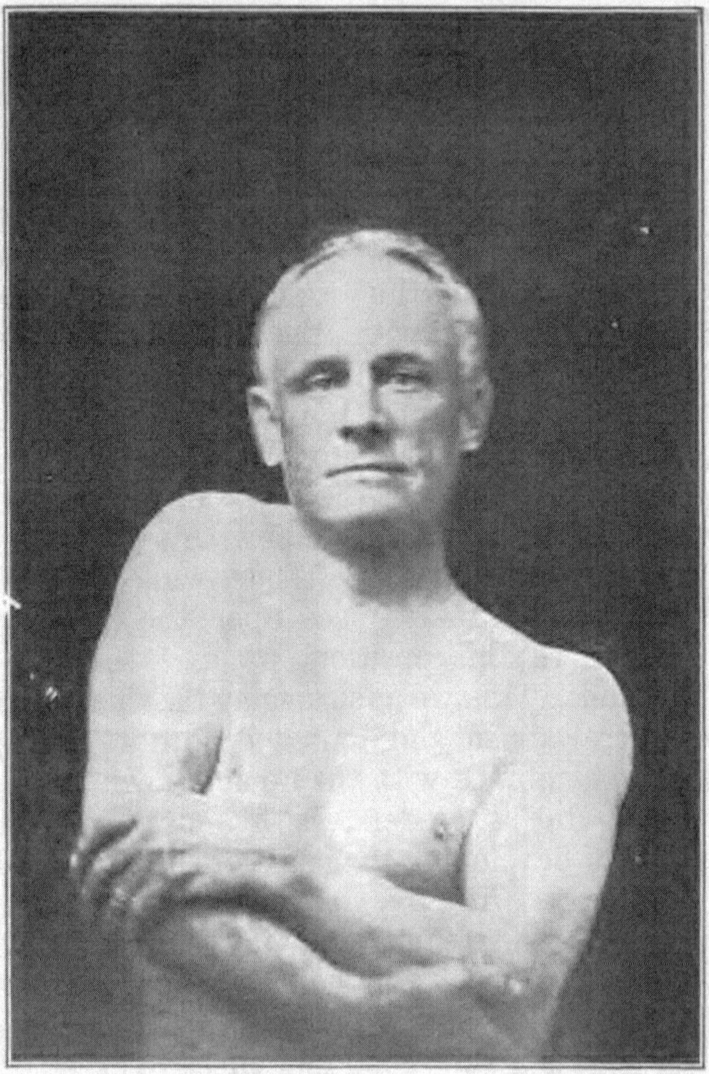

Developing the Muscles of the Shoulder Blades

Exercise for Developing the Muscles Covering the Shoulder Blades

LYING upon your back, alternately raise your shoulders, as shown in the illustration on the opposite page. The tension should be upward and forward as far as possible.

Commence with five movements upon each side; it is perfectly safe, and in a very short time all feeling of soreness, which may result from the first attempts, will disappear. The movements can then be increased without fatigue, and with very satisfactory results, to ten times the original number.

By reference to the anatomical plate on page 316, you will see that this movement will bring into action the large muscles attached to, and covering, the shoulder blades. It is an excellent exercise for ladies who may be deficient at this point, improvement being certain if these directions are faithfully followed. If your shoulders were ever well developed and symmetrical, that condition can certainly be restored by persistent practice of this exercise.

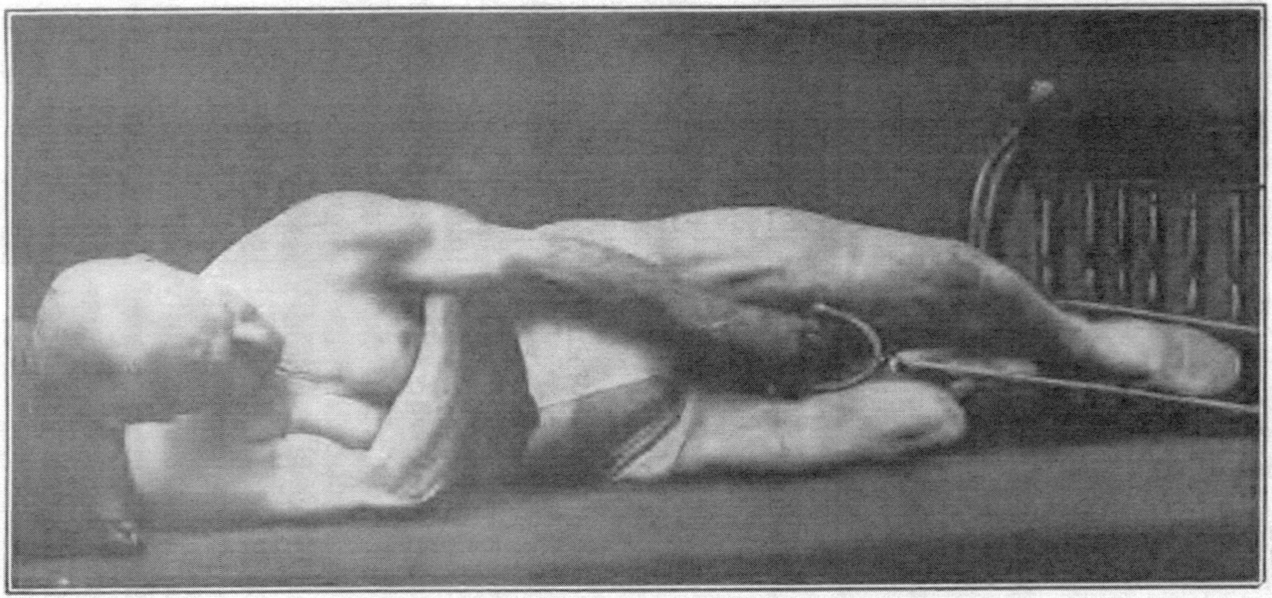

Developing the "Climbing Muscles"

Exercise for the Development of the Legs

The Climbing Muscles

IN most persons the legs, as they are constantly exercised in the ordinary pursuits of life, are proportionately better developed than the arms. But the mere exercise of walking will not specially develop the large muscles at the front of the thighs and in the calves of the legs, which I will designate as the "climbing muscles." Walking or running, while either brings those muscles into action, does not place any considerable tension upon them, and as a rule neither pedestrians nor fast runners are notable for any unusual development at these points; while, on the other hand, bicyclists and "men of the hills" are almost invariably well developed there.

The leg muscles of the runner are more elastic, and capable of more rapid action, than are those of the adept of the silent wheel or the athlete of the hills, but the former soon tires under the strain of a steady climb, whatever his physical condition may be, simply because he has not developed the muscles then called into action.

It is really only a matter of training. My attention was called to this marked deficiency in the cases of several well-known runners and pedestrians, members of a celebrated San Francisco athletic club. Upon several occasions these gentlemen were the guests of an outing club to which I belonged for several years. We owned a small pack of fox hounds with which we were in the habit of hunting coyotes. The country in which we hunted is very rough, hilly, and impracticable for horses; we therefore followed the hounds on foot.

A coyote, when chased by hounds, always selects for his line of flight the roughest country he can find; and to cut off his flight usually meant a running climb over hills too steep and high to be available for anything but pasturage for the half-wild cattle wandering over them. If the run led up a valley or over level country our guests had no trouble in jogging on ahead of us, apparently as tireless as the hounds whose wild chorus echoed through the canyon; but when the scrub wolf changed his course, and started over the "high divide," the conditions changed. The elastic muscles of the athletes, accustomed only to the smooth floor of the gymnasium or the level cinder path, quickly tired when called upon to face the steep sides of "rocky ridge."

I have seen one of these gentlemen make a good showing in a five-mile flat race, while another once held a low mark at 220 yards, and at the time in question both were in excellent condition. But the steep grade and the steady strain of the "high divide," while but a jog for the slower men who were accustomed to the climb, were too much for them.

This, or any other athletic feat, is not so much a matter of natural ability, as of the training of the muscles specially brought into play by the exertion.

The development of these "climbing muscles" of the legs for any exercise of this nature will interest very few, but as a means of developing and adding to the symmetry of the legs, it is very possible that the simple and effective means I will suggest may be of more general interest. To bring into action the large muscles on the front of the thigh and those that make up the calf of the leg, *i. e.*, the "climbing muscles," it is necessary to exert a pressure upon the ball of the foot, which can be accomplished very easily as you lie in bed.

Attach to the foot of your bed a cord about 1½ feet in length, terminating in a pulley weight handle. Lying upon your side, grasp this handle, then press firmly against the footboard of the bed with the ball of the foot, and alternately relax the pressure. This alternate pressure and relaxation will actively exercise the muscles in question, will imitate the action of climbing with the leg so exercised, and will bring no strain or possible injury upon the heart —a danger ever imminent in hill climbing.

The pressure exerted should be equal to that required in climbing stairs or a steep grade. This exercise, if persistently and regularly practiced, will surely improve the symmetry of the legs, and will give one an ability to ascend stairs or climb steep hills, which can never be acquired by the same amount of walking or ordinary gymnasium running exercise. It should be practiced upon both the left and the right side; otherwise the development will be unequal. (See illustration, page 338).

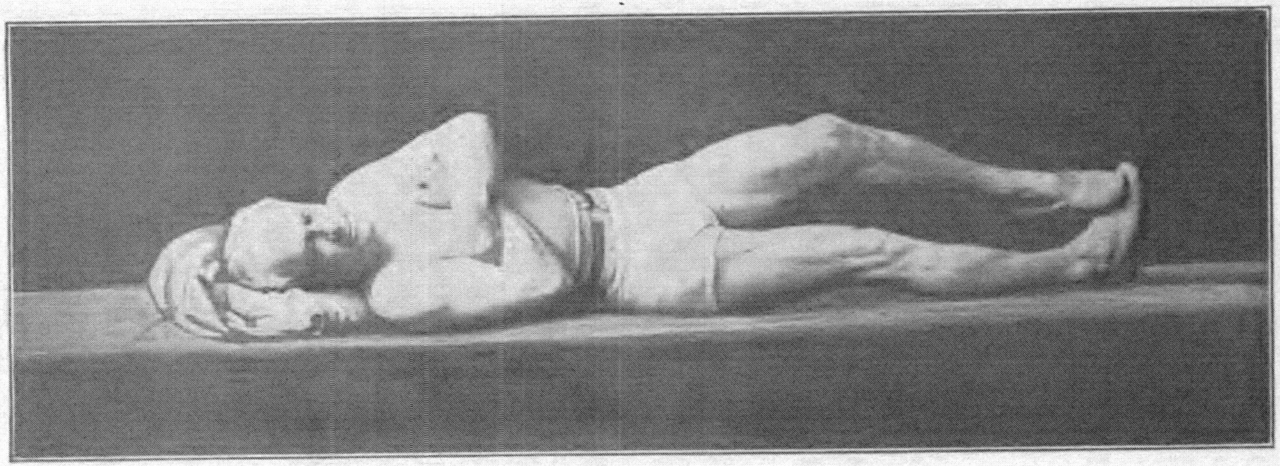

The Climbing Muscles—Exercise No. 2

Development of the Muscles of the Legs

(Continued)

If from any circumstances the cord and pulley weight handle described in the foregoing chapter should be found inconvenient, simply rest the ball of the foot against the footboard of the bed and alternately press and relax; or still another and easier way—lying upon your back or partially upon the side, as shown in the accompanying illustration, place the ball of the left foot upon the upper part or toes of the right, tense the muscles of this right leg and foot so that it may afford support, then alternately press and relax with the left foot. Repeat the exercise with the other leg.

The cord and pulley weight handle device is far more effective and development is quicker, but the last two exercises as described can be practiced under all circumstances and will appeal to the members of the greatest organization on earth; *i. e.*, lazy people, of which the writer is a member and a good example.

For this reason all of these exercises are designed to get the greatest amount of special muscular activity with as little general exertion as possible. It is a lazy man's system, but you will find that any and all of these exercises are remarkably effective.

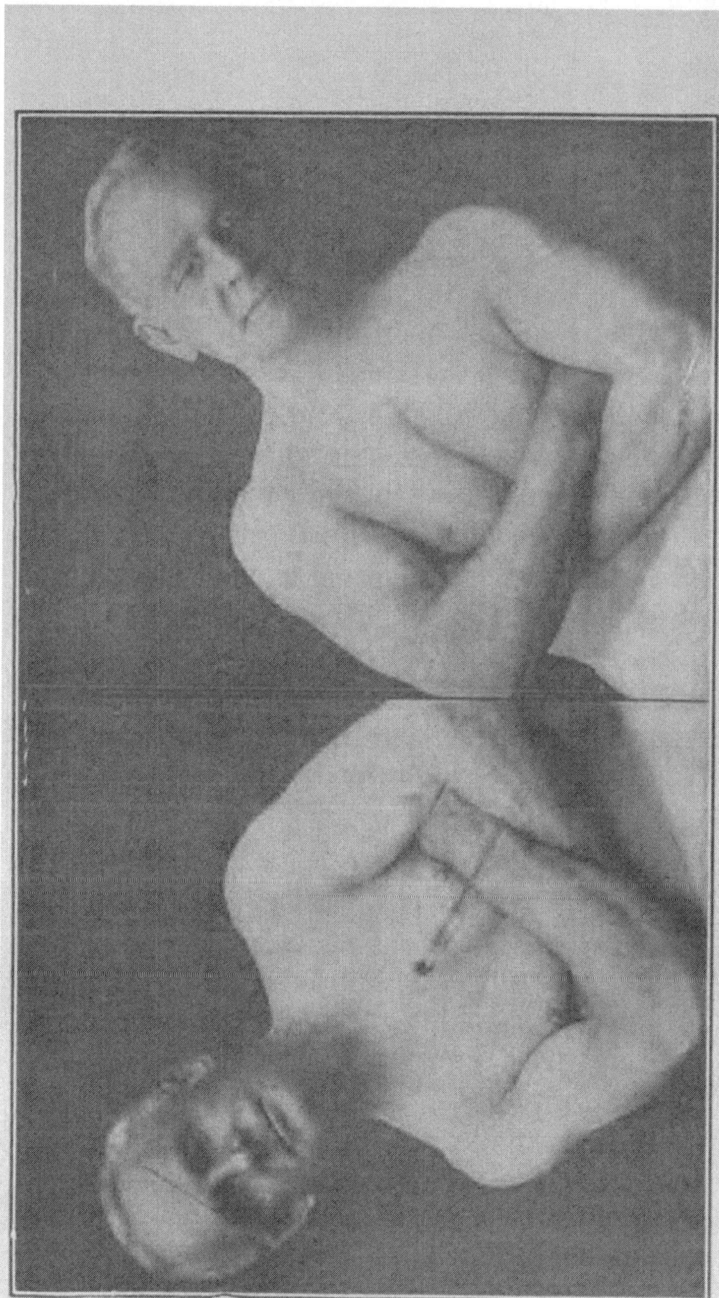

Developing the Loin Muscles

Exercise for Strengthening the Loins

IN that system of military drill familiarly known as the "setting-up drill," there is an exercise especially designed for the development of the loins and side muscles. Standing erect, with the hands upon the hips, the men bend the upper part of the body as far to one side as possible; then reverse, bending to the other side, thus alternately tensing and relaxing the muscles of the loins. It is an excellent method of strengthening the body at this point, as well as a remedy for constipation.

This exercise can be easily performed while lying in bed.

Resting upon your back, with your arms folded across the chest, raise the head and shoulders slightly, so as to clear the pillow.

Commence with ten movements; that is, five upon each side; as your physical condition improves, increase to twenty-five.

This action will tense the abdominal muscles, and place a moderate tension upon the loin muscles, the weight of the head and shoulders being an excellent substitute for the mechanical appliances sometimes used. In combination with, and following, the exercise with the lifting board, every muscle of the loins and sides will be brought into healthy action. If faithfully and systematically practiced, improvement is certain. (See illustration on page 345.)

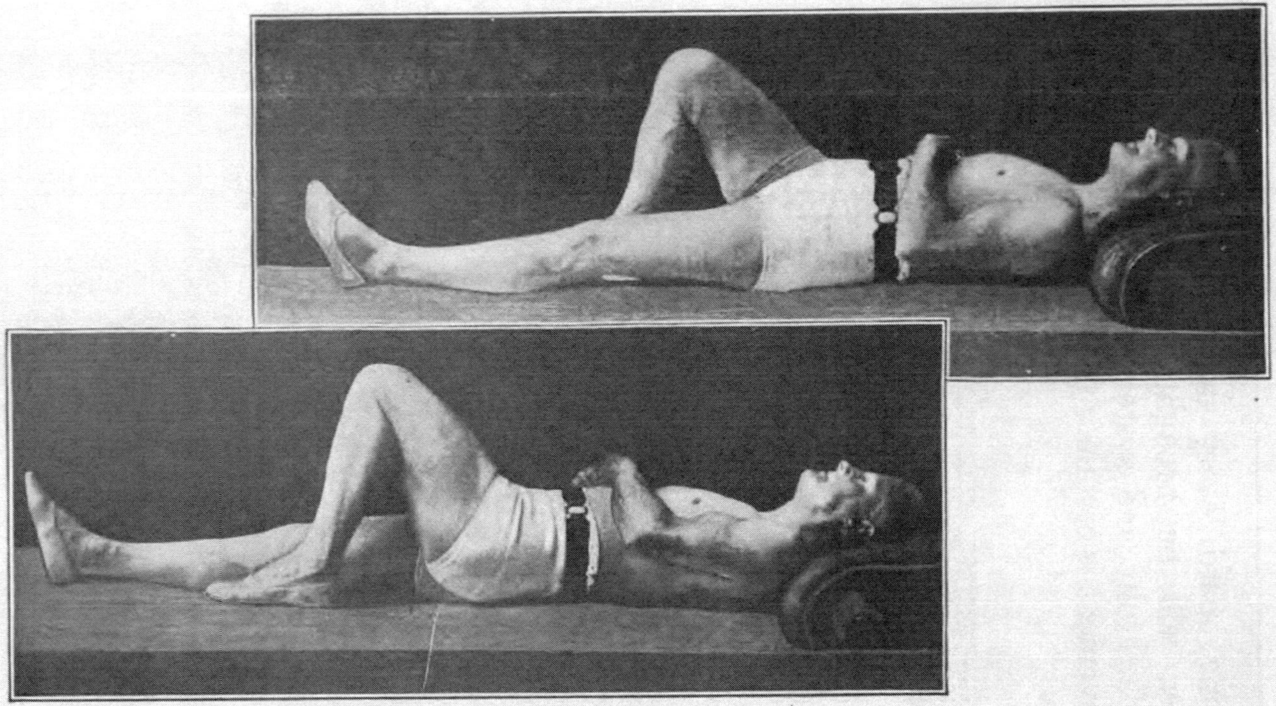

Developing the Lower Abdominal Muscles

Exercise for Strengthening the Lower Abdominal Muscles

IN the human being the lower abdominal muscles, which cover that part of the abdomen lying between the hips and lower portion of the pelvic bones, are subject to a continuous strain, as they support the heavy viscera within. If they become weakened through inaction they will relax, and that unsightly condition known as "pot bellied" may result. A far greater danger is also ever present; the possibility—really the probability—of rupture from any sudden strain.

A brief description of these muscles will enable you to understand more clearly the following exercise, designed for strengthening these muscles.

The external, or descending, oblique muscles are situated on the side and fore-part of the abdomen. They are the largest and most superficial of the broad, thin, flat muscles that brace and support the lower part of the abdomen. They are firmly attached to the external surface and lower borders of the inferior, or lower, ribs. From these cartilaginous attachments other smaller muscles proceed in various directions. They lap, overlap, and interlace, and thus form a muscular webbing designed to support and protect the underlying bowels and organs. These external muscles are again braced by a system of deep-seated internal muscles, the whole forming a wonderfully ingenious structure designed to support and protect the underlying organs.

At this part of the body great muscular strength is requisite to sustain the pressure of the viscera within. If these muscles become weakened, serious results may follow.

The importance of especially exercising and strengthening these supporting muscles is therefore evident. This is very difficult to accomplish when standing erect, but can be readily effected in a recumbent position, as follows:

Lying upon your back, as shown in the illustration on page 348, bend one knee upwards and inwards; as you do so, draw up the hip of that side. You will find this action tenses all of the lower abdominal muscles. Then drop that leg back to its original position, and bend the knee, and draw up the hip of the other side. Alternate in the exercising, first upon the right side, then the left.

The illustration shows the knee bent more than may be necessary, as after a few trials you will acquire control of the hip movement, after which the exercise will be very easy and improvement rapid.

Commence with three movements upon each side, increasing, as your physical condition improves, to twenty-five.

This exercise is valuable in cases of constipation; and when the muscles described are toned up and strengthened, rupture is a very remote possibility.

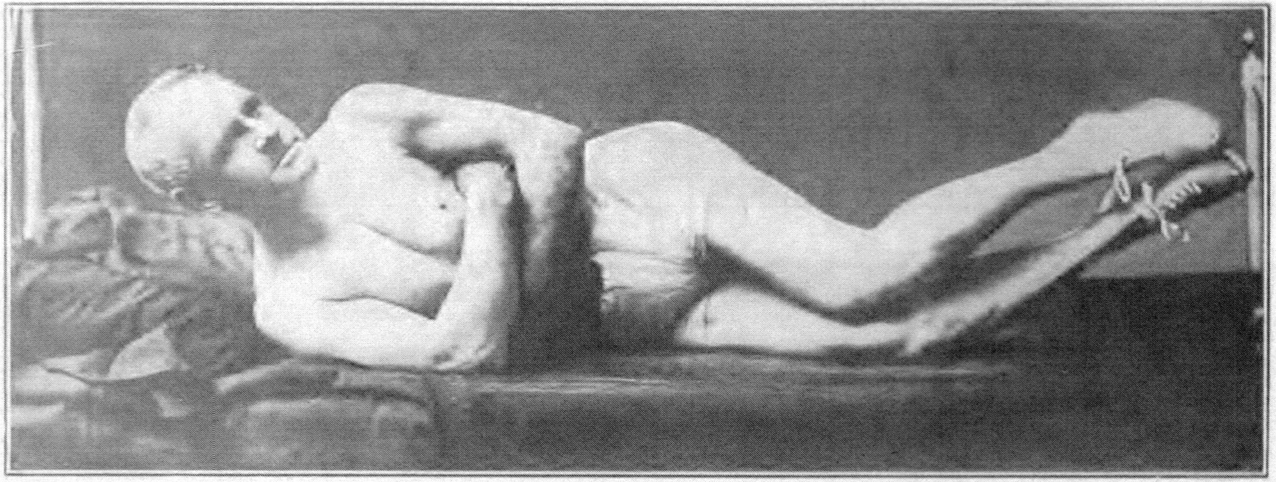

Muscles of the Sides. 5 Movements

Exercise for Developing the Muscles of the Sides and Loins

LYING upon your side, as shown in the illustration on the opposite page, raise the head and both feet at once; this will contract the side muscles of the loins and the large muscles which descend from immediately below the arm pits into the loins. The exercise will also strengthen the muscles of the stomach. It is an excellent one, but somewhat fatiguing.

Commence with but three movements. Six or seven will probably prove the limit to which you will care to go, as the strain is equivalent to lifting a heavy weight by the muscles described. Therefore, if adopted, the exercise must be commenced and practiced with caution.

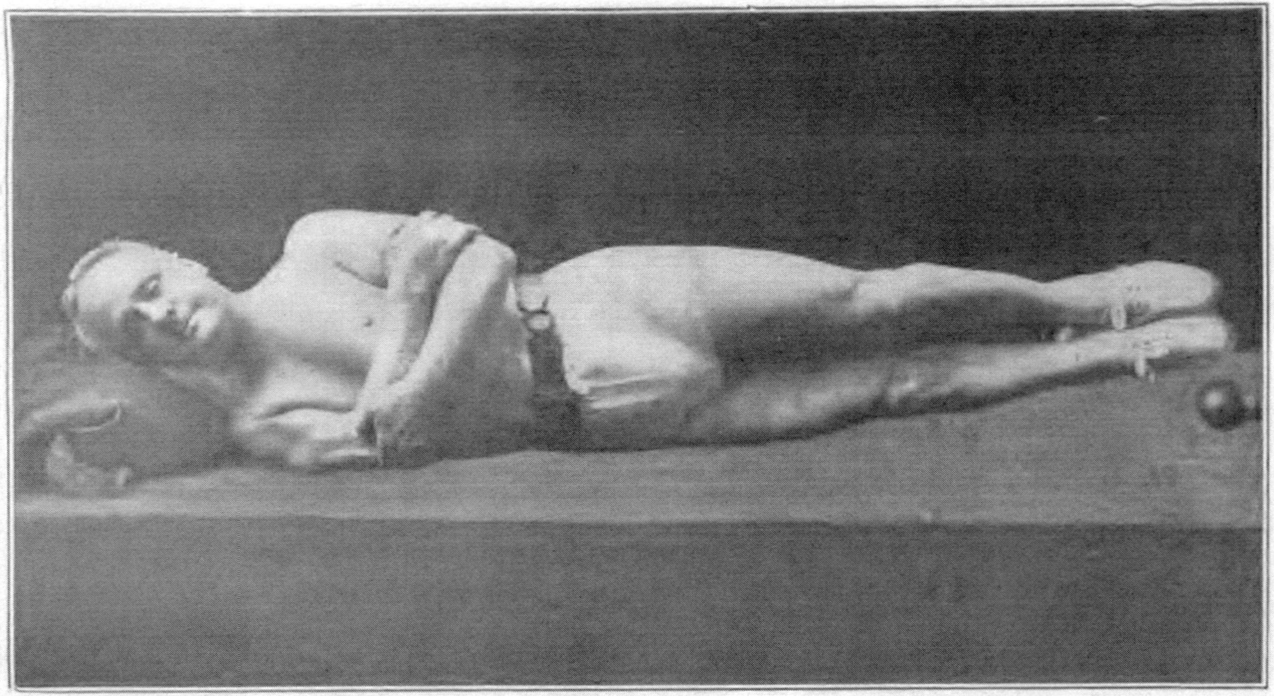

Developing the Whole Body by Tensing

Tensing Exercise for the Whole Body

THERE are many deep-seated minor muscles which are not called into activity by the special exercises previously described. The capillaries which should nourish them, and the microscopic veins, by this inactivity, may become clogged, losing their elasticity and efficiency, just as the larger arteries, veins and muscles will deteriorate under like conditions. It is therefore necessary to bring this dormant machinery into action. To effect this, lie upon your side, fold your arms across your chest, grasp your elbows with the hands, throw your head well back, and stretch your body to its full length, as shown in the illustration upon the opposite page. In this attitude exert at first but half of the strength of your folded arms—the pressure coming upon the elbows, over which your hands are clasped. As you do this, stretch and tense your entire body until it becomes rigid. Hold this position but two or three seconds, as the effect is as though you were lifting a heavy weight. Relax for a few seconds; then repeat the effort. Three or four movements—that is, alternate tensing and relaxing of the muscles

—as described are sufficient. This exercise will set the blood "tingling in every vein," and, most probably, will be followed at first by perspiration.

Commence the exercise cautiously; exert only half your force in the pressure of the folded arms, and gradually increase, as your strength increases. Commence with not more than three or four movements; increase slowly until you have reached ten, which will be sufficient.

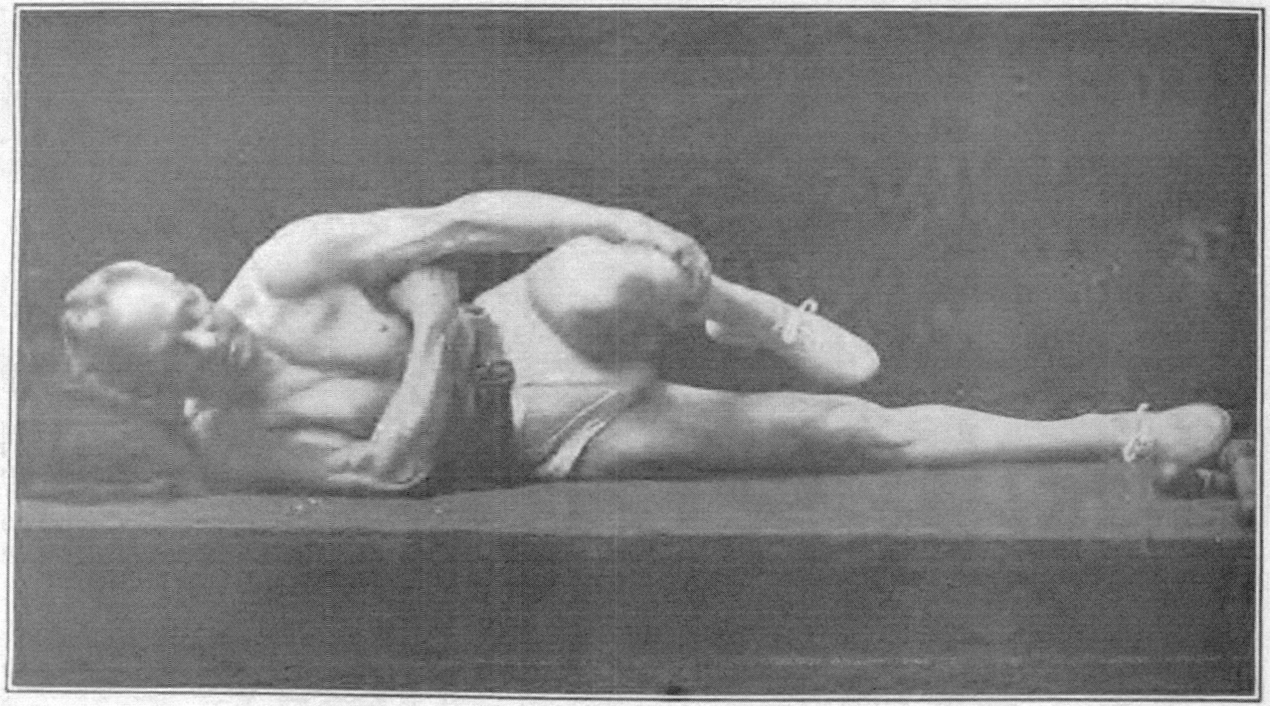

Developing the Back and Loins by Single-Arm Pulling Exercise

Single-Arm Pulling Exercise

LYING upon your side, as in the preceding exercise, clasp one hand only around the ankle of the upper leg, as in the illustration on preceding page. In this position, pull with your full strength, holding the strain for a few seconds; then relax.

Commence with ten movements (that is, alternately tensing and relaxing by the pulling exercise described), and increase, as your physical condition improves, to twenty-five movements.

You will find the tension of the shoulder muscles in this effort different from the preceding exercise, the strain being across the shoulders as well as downward. This, like the pulling exercise, is perfectly safe; the muscles specially brought into action are those which make up the "neck yoke" and those immediately around and bracing the shoulder sockets. It is designed to strengthen and generally develop the muscles of the back.

Pulling Exercise, for Strengthening the Muscles of the Back and Loins

LYING upon your side, clasp your hands over the upper knee, as shown in the illustration on following page. Exert your full strength in a steady pull; then relax.

Commence with ten movements (that is, alternately pulling steadily a few seconds upon the bent knee and then relaxing the strain). As you gain strength, increase the movements.

The tension will come principally upon the back muscles of the shoulders, but this is also an excellent exercise for the development of the loin muscles, which are brought into action by the effort.

This exercise is perfectly safe, and improvement in the muscles so treated is certain, if the exercise is systematically and regularly practiced.

In all of these exercises, when the position is upon the side, go through the whole series for that side before changing the position. I practice in the order of the descriptions and illustrations.

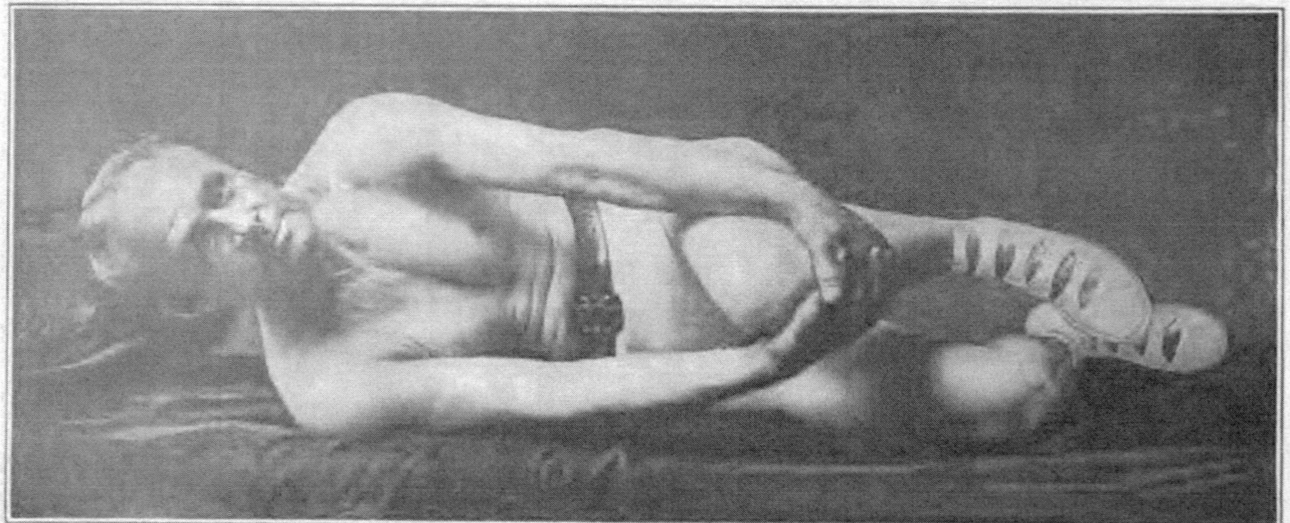

Developing the Back and Loins by Pulling Exercise

Exercise for Developing the Back and Shoulder Muscles

IN this exercise, remain in the same position as that just described—that is, upon your side, with the arms folded across the chest—bend the head well forward, thus tensing the muscles at the base of the neck, and those surrounding it. Exert your full strain upon the folded arms (the lower part of the body being relaxed); in this position shrug your shoulders up and down. This action will alternately tense and relax the large muscles of the upper part of the neck and shoulders.

Commence with five movements, and increase to, say, fifteen.

This is a very effective exercise, and is without danger of strain.

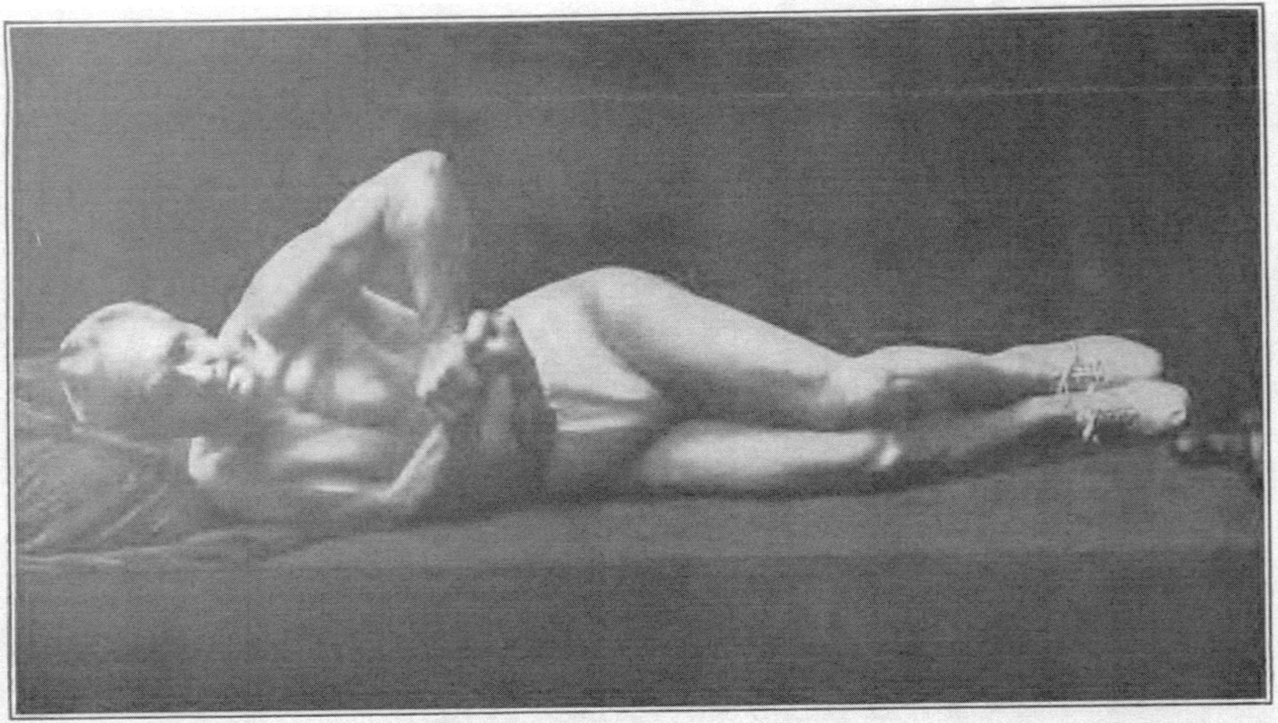

Developing the Fore-Arms by Resistance

Resistance Exercise for Developing the Fore-Arms

LYING upon your side, grasp the wrist of your lower arm with the upper hand; press with your full strength downward, resisting with upward pressure, as in the illustration on the opposite page.

Commence with five movements; that is, alternately exerting and relaxing the pressure upon the lower wrist; increase as your physical condition improves, to ten or fifteen. It is a perfectly safe exercise, and will add to the strength of the fore-arm.

This exercise is specially designed for the development of the fore-arm, but you will find that it brings into action and tenses all the muscles of the arm. It should be practiced both upon the right and left side. (See illustration on opposite page.)

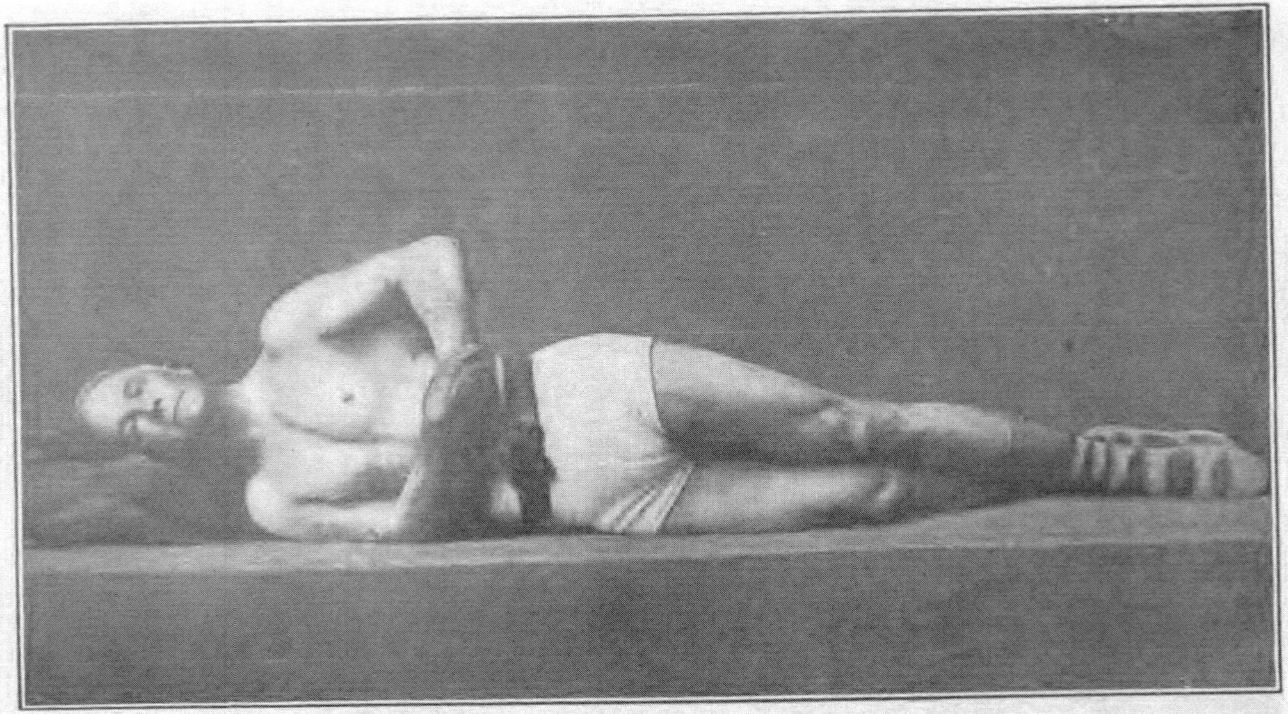

Developing the Arms by Resistance

Resistance Exercise for Developing the Arms

LYING upon your side, as shown in the illustration on the opposite page, grasp the upper wrist with the lower hand and pull upward with the upper arm, resisting that pull with the downward strain of the lower arm. At each movement, that is, in the alternate strain and relaxation of the muscles, turn the wrist slightly, as it lies in the clasp of the hand. In the one position, the front of the wrist should meet the palm of the opposing hand; and in the next, the side of the wrist should be presented to it.

This slight change, made by the turn of the wrist, will bring into action another set of muscles, and if you desire to thoroughly exercise the muscular system, do not overlook these apparently trivial changes in position.

To ladies endeavoring to improve the symmetry of their arms, I strongly recommend this exercise. Commence with ten movements, and increase, as your physical condition improves, even to the point of fatigue. Benefit will surely result.

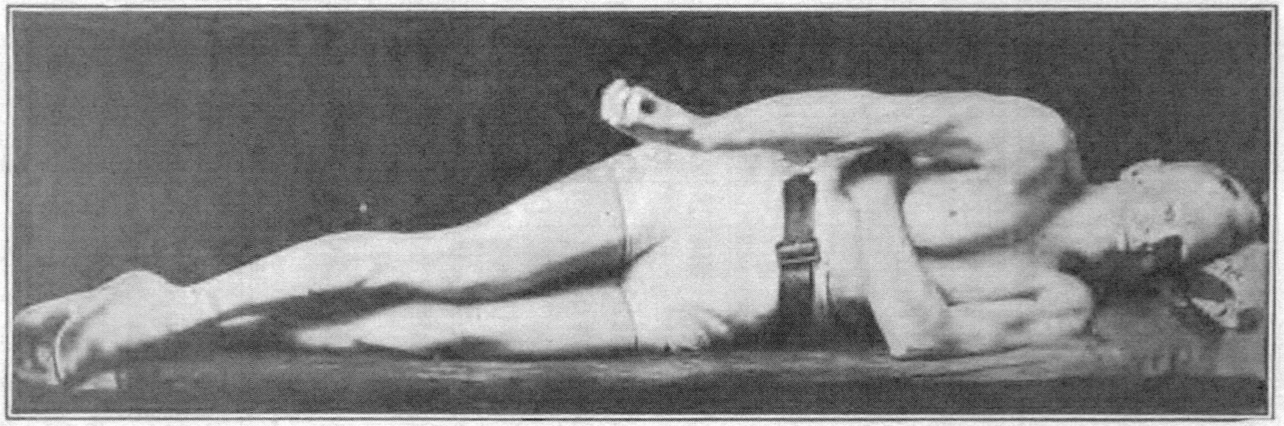

Developing the Arm by Twisting Exercise

Twisting Exercise for the Development of the Arms

THIS movement brings into action all the muscles of the arms, and is exactly like the exercise of fencing, in which the play of the foils necessitates this twisting motion. The benefits of fencing are well known; but as only the right arm is used by the fencer in his amusement that arm is often unduly developed, while the left is neglected. He is, therefore, in this respect, usually ill-balanced.

In lying upon your side, extend your upper arm at full length, parallel with your body, as shown in the illustration facing this page. Clench your fist tightly, that the muscles may be tensed. Twist your arm around toward your body as far as possible without inconvenience; then reverse the movement.

Commence with five or ten movements; that is, twisting the arm backward an dforward, as directed.

This is an excellent exercise for ladies who wish to add to the symmetry of their arms, as improvement is certain if the practice is persistent. It is, of course, understood that both the right arm and the left must be exercised in this manner; otherwise an unequal development will surely result.

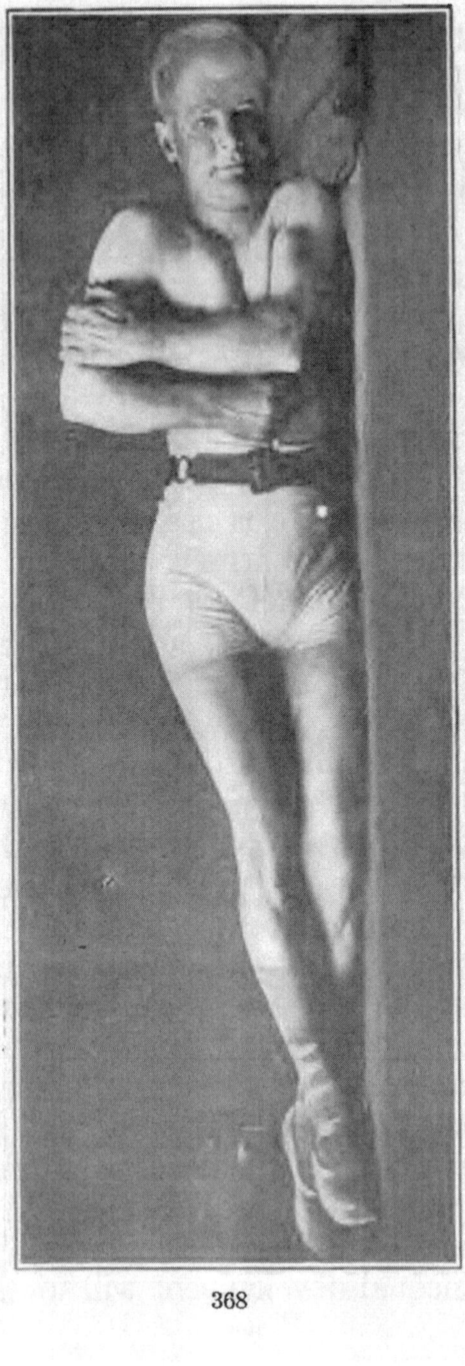

Developing the Back Muscles of the Arms

Exercise for Developing the Triceps or Back Muscles of the Arms

LYING upon your side, grasp firmly the upper arm, between the elbow and the shoulder, as in the position shown in the illustration facing this page. Pull backwards with the upper arm, at the same time resisting the pull by the firm grasp and downward pull of the lower hand and arm.

Commence with five movements; that is, alternately pulling and relaxing the strain.

I do not know of any gymnasium exercise, aided by mechanical appliances, that will so speedily develop the muscles described. It is a safe, simple and very effective exercise.

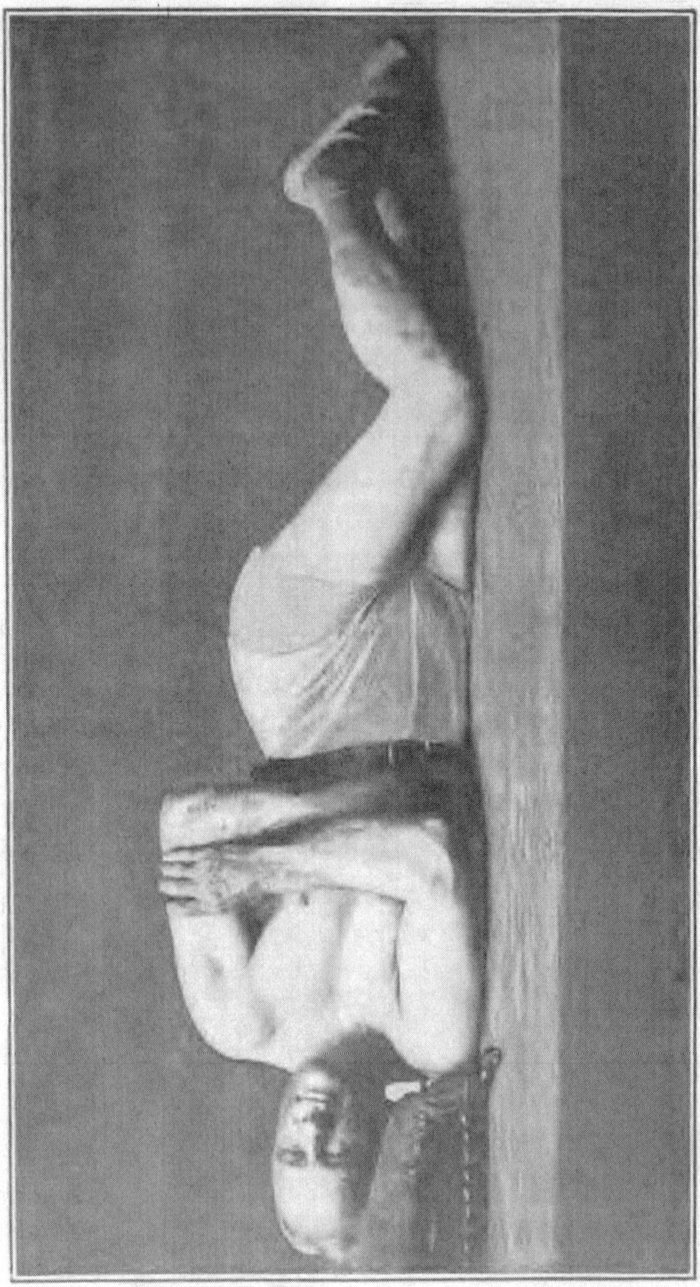

Exercise for Hip and Loins

Exercise for the Hips and Loins

LYING upon your side throw the upper hip forward, as in the illustration. As you do so bend your arm and draw it back as far as possible. This action will place an additional tension upon the loin muscles, as well as upon the muscles of the contracted arm. Relax and repeat. Three to five movements will be sufficient to commence with, but as you increase in strength, double that number will not fatigue and will be of benefit. This is an excellent and perfectly safe exercise. It will strengthen and give elasticity to the loin muscles. It also brings the abdominal muscles into action. The movement of the upper hip should be simultaneous with the back movement of the elbow. In the picture the lower hand is shown to be grasping the upper arm, but this I no longer practice, as I have found that it interferes with the forward hip movement, which can then not be extended as far forward as if the hand were free in the exercise. It is true that it has a beneficial effect upon the muscles of the contracted upper arm, but as I have said I now practice with the upper arm free. Practice upon both sides of the body.

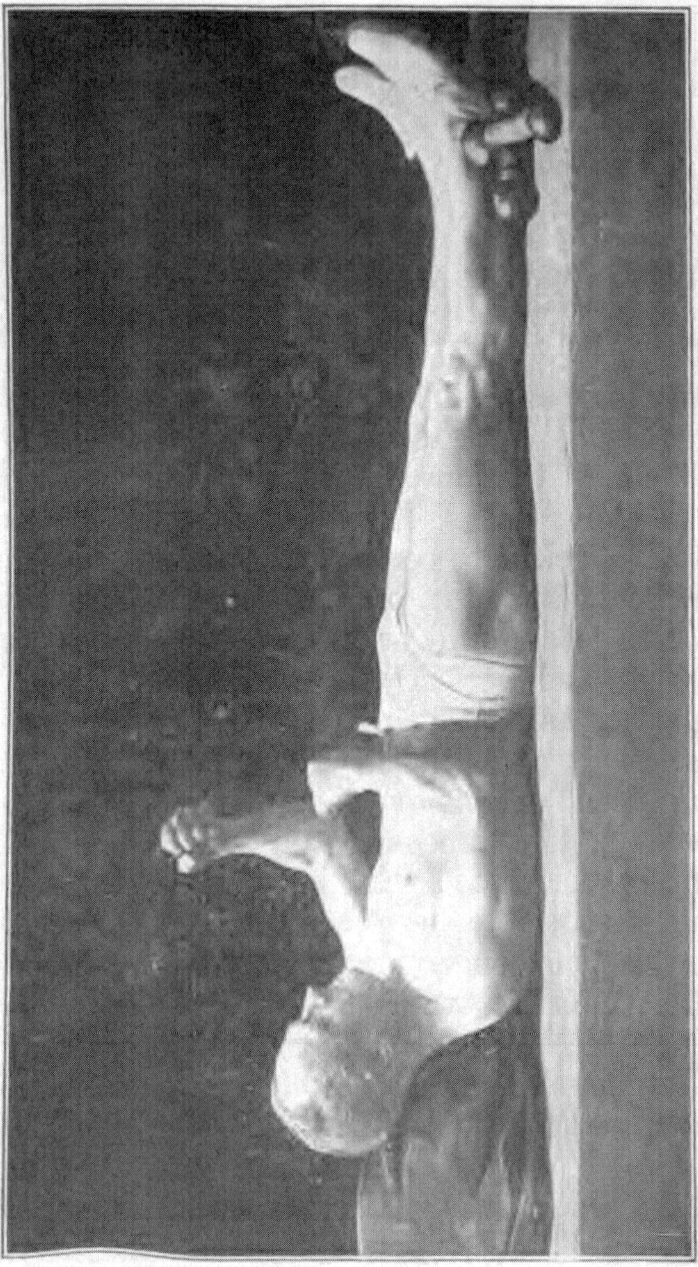

Developing the Abdominal Muscles by Percussion

Percussion Exercise for Strengthening the Abdominal Muscles and Improving Digestion

THIS method of exercise is described in the pages headed "Dyspepsia." There is but little to add to that statement. Suffice it, then, to say that it is an excellent exercise, and has a very beneficial effect upon all the digestive organs.

Commence with twenty-five quick strokes; increase, as your physical condition will warrant, to one hundred or more. The percussion should be light and rapid.

Continue the percussion, both in the tensed and relaxed conditions of the abdominal muscles, as produced in the foregoing exercise; the tension and relaxation being caused by alternately raising and lowering the head, as in the illustration on the opposite page.

During intervals of rest, if it is desired to reduce the abdominal fat, massage and rub the fatty deposit as directed upon the page headed "Reducing an Obese Abdomen." If you find you are impeded by the bedclothes, bend the knees, which will raise the covering clear of the abdomen.

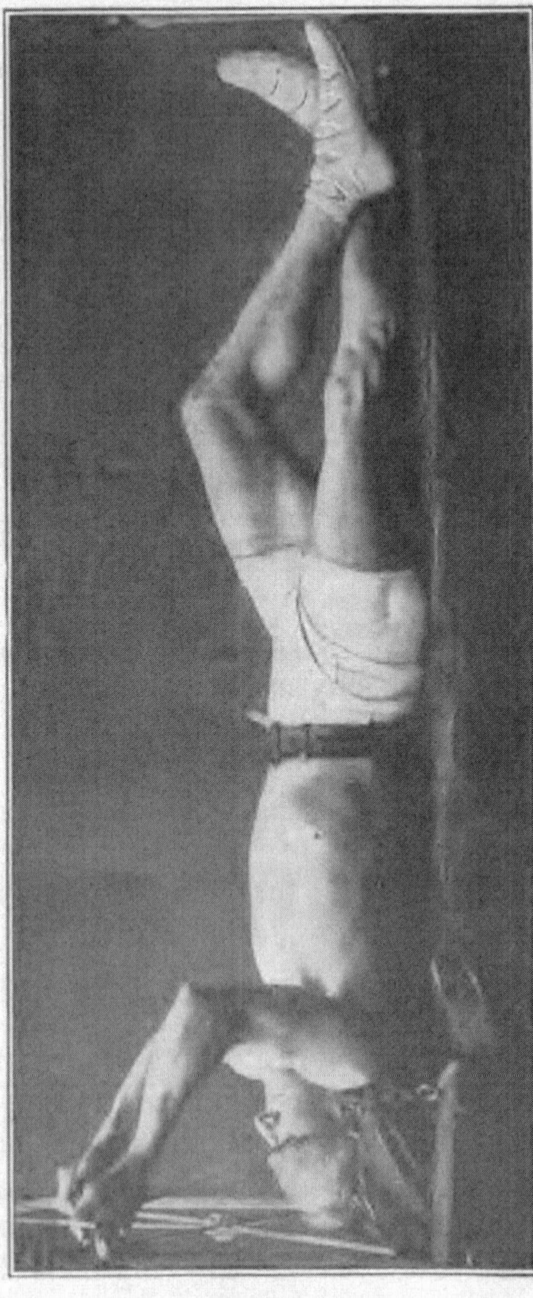

Developing the Arms and Shoulders by Bar Exercise Number 1

Bar Exercise No. 1

Exercise Number 1 for the Development of the Muscles of the Arms and Shoulders

FIRMLY attached across the head-board of my bed is a stout hickory bar 1½ inches in diameter and as long as the head-board is wide.

Lying upon my back, I grasp this bar with both hands, as shown in the illustration on the opposite page. I employ sufficient strength to bring the muscles of my arms to full tension, but not to move the body.

Commence the exercise with five motions; increase gradually, until your physical condition will warrant twenty-five daily without fatigue or soreness of the muscles.

I weigh, stripped, 140 pounds; the force of the pull would not raise more than half of that weight, therefore the body moves but slightly from its position, while the muscles of the arms and shoulders are thoroughly exercised.

The method I have described is perfectly safe at any age; the pull can be proportioned to your physical condition and the heart will not be overtaxed.

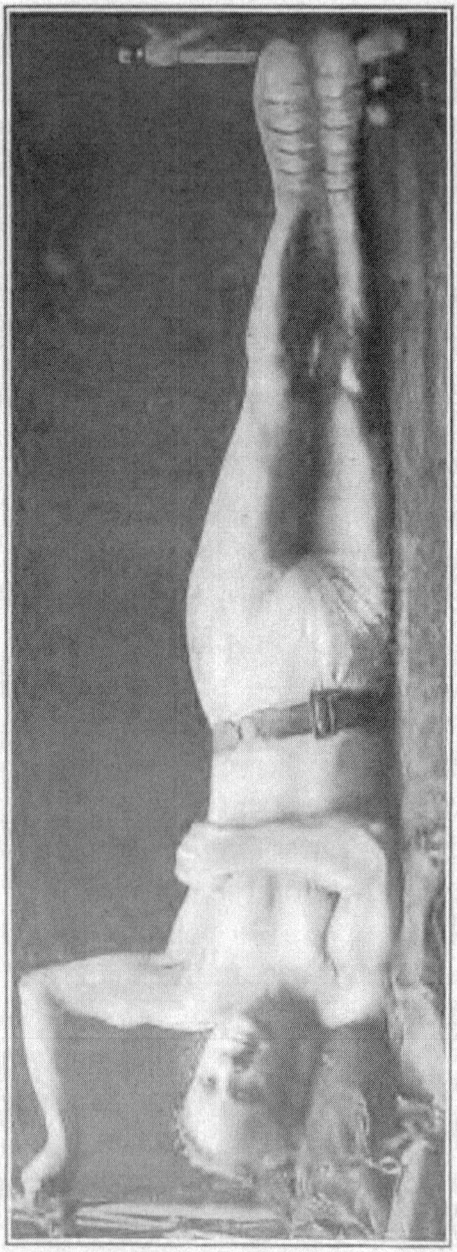

Developing the Arms and Shoulders by Bar Exercise Number 2

Bar Exercise Number 2

Similar to the Foregoing Exercise, with the Exception that but One Hand Is Used

THIS exercise is designed to stretch the large muscles immediately surrounding, and below, the arm pit, which do not seem to be so directly called into action when using both arms. The shoulder, in this exercise, is raised higher, and the tension upon the muscles described is more decided. See anatomical plate, facing page 34.

Commence with five movements and gradually increase to twenty-five, as your physical condition may warrant. (Exercise illustrated on opposite page.)

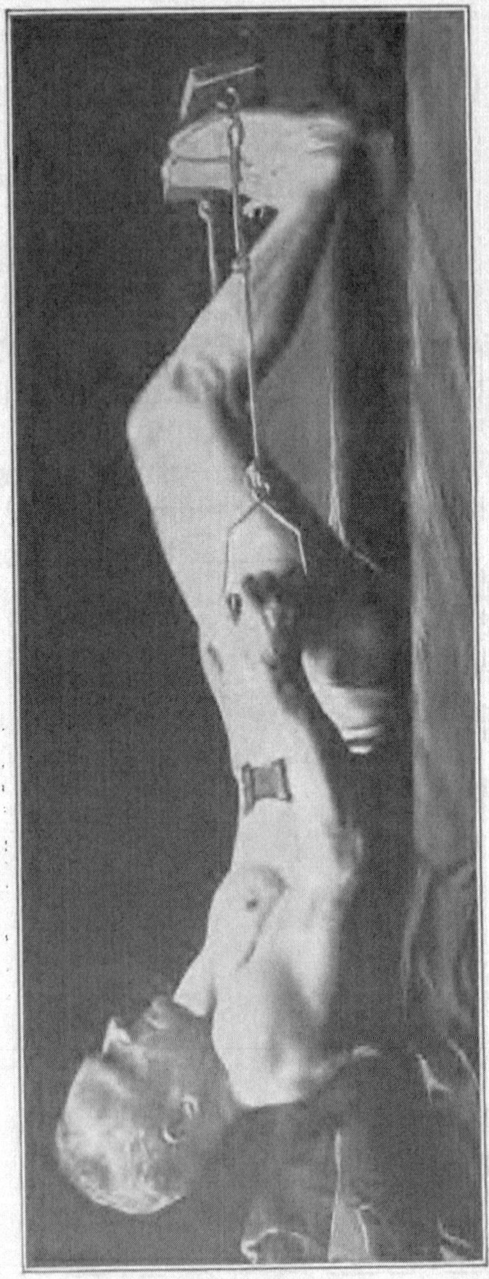

Using the Lifting Board

The Lifting Board

THIS exercise was devised in response to many inquiries from athletes who desired some simple substitute for the ordinary expensive lifting machine used in gymnasiums—something which could be used in connection with this comfortable system of exercises.

The answer to these inquiries is this lifting board. It will be found an excellent device for developing the muscles called into action in weight-lifting, but is not necessary to those whose object in taking up this system is simply health. To the athlete I strongly advocate the use of this device, but in moderation. A very marked increase in your weight-lifting ability will soon appear, but practice in moderation.

This simple but very effective device for exercising the muscles of the shoulders and loins and thighs is a board 15 inches in length by 4 inches in width. At each end are inserted two strong screw eyes, to which are attached ropes 18 inches long, terminating in ordinary pulley-weight handles. This board is covered with flannel, to prevent a chill to the feet.

The method of its use is shown by the

illustration on page 378; the effect is that of the ordinary lifting machine, with the advantage that it is used in a recumbent position, and under cover of the bed-clothes. It is the only exercise I describe in which there is any danger of injury, as it is possible to strain the muscles of the loins or shoulders, if too great force is exerted; therefore, in commencing the practice, put on the strain gently for a few seconds; then relax. This alternate tension and relaxation by the lifting movement specially brings into action the muscles of the shoulders, loins and thighs; but it is also an excellent exercise for the whole body.

The apparatus is very simple and easily made. Do not use springs or elastic bands, which you will be tempted to do, thinking they are an improvement. I used them and abandoned them in favor of the inflexible ropes.

The elasticity of the loin muscles in the act of lifting will be sufficient, and you will be better able to determine the amount of lifting strain required. I strongly advocate this exercise, but in moderation. Commence with five gentle movements, increasing, as strength develops, and your physical condition may warrant.

Man's First Physical Culture System

IT is evident that the lazy but logical methods of muscular activity I have so successfully practiced, appeal to a great many other lazy people, both men and women, old or young. Yet my simple methods of physical culture, as described in "Old Age—Its Cause and Prevention," are not new. All healthy babies practice exercises something similar; *i. e.,* as they lie in their cradles, cribs or mothers' arms. You practiced the same exercises when you were a baby, and babies will continue to practice this system of physical culture as long as human beings inhabit this earth, for in the squirms, contortions and increasing activity of healthy infants, you will see Nature's methods of developing their muscular structure. So I will confess that I simply stole this system of exercise from these immature men and women.

For the rapid changes of position of the little mite of humanity (made all in a few minutes) see illustrations upon pages 382 and 383. You may say that if you had baby's elastic arteries and normally rapid heart action, you, too, could exercise as fast without danger. To understand this statement, turning to page 198 and looking

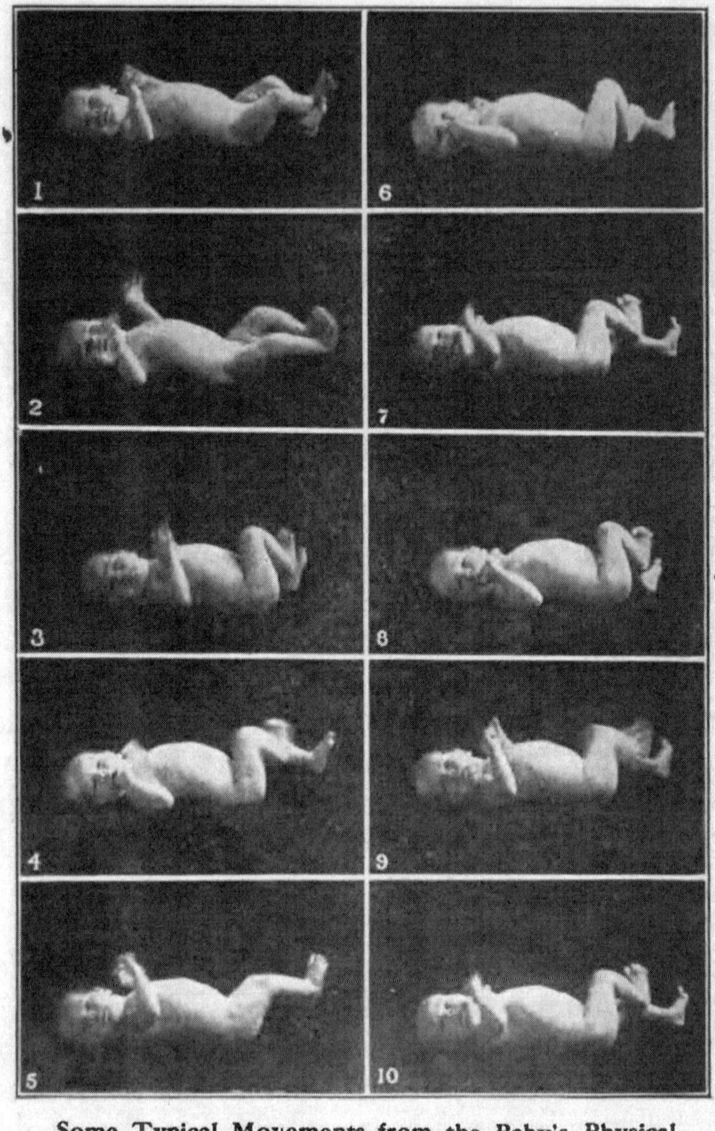

Some Typical Movements from the Baby's Physical Culture System

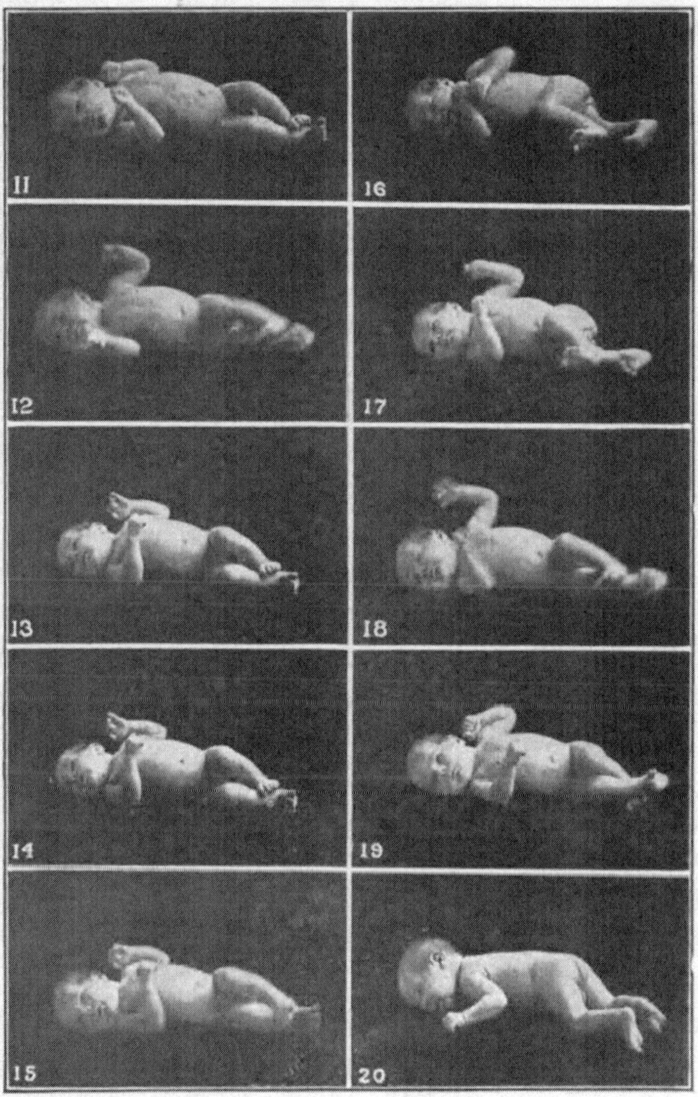

An Additional Series of Movements Typical of Baby's Natural System of Exercise

over Prof. W. F. Porter's table of "Pulse Frequency" there given, note the great difference between your pulsations and those of a baby one year old. I will assume you are between 55 and 60. Your normal pulse at those ages would rate along at about 75, while baby's normal heart beat would be 134; that is during its infrequent periods of quiet; and when it was in activity, which would be nearly all the time, it would probably rise to 150 or more. In my exercises I am continually testing my pulse; indeed, I have become so accustomed to doing this that a touch of my finger upon my wrist for only two or three pulsations is all that I need to keep well within a safe rate. This pulse-testing is easily acquired; learn exactly where to find the pulsation in your wrist, and the test can be quickly made. You do not need a watch, as you will speedily determine the approximate rate by a touch, three or four pulsations, as I have said, being amply sufficient. About 80 would be a good, slow exercising pulse, but five or six beats faster, under those conditions would probably be safe enough. You will find that when you awake, and before exercising, the rate will be say 10 or 12 beats slower—at least it should be.

Regarding baby's exercises: upon the following pages I present twenty instantaneous photographs of the different positions assumed by a healthy three weeks' old baby taken during the ten minutes this active little mite was under the sensitive eye of the camera. Thirty-eight snapshots were made, but as many seemed to be but repetitions of some preceding movement, I have used only those which show some variation of position.

Therefore, practice the exercises described and illustrated in this book, but practice them slowly.

As to the time of practice—commence as soon as you are awake, and before you rise. If you are unable to sleep, and you toss and tumble, and hear the clock strike all kinds of uncanny hours, don't bother counting imaginary sheep or employing other standard methods of inducing sleep, but select any one of the exercises I describe, preferably one of the arm exercises which requires as little movement as possible. Practice this very slowly, so slowly that it may become monotonous, also slightly fatiguing, and count the movements very deliberately, as in the time-honored practice of counting sheep, jumping over a fence; start—one—two—three, etc., until you are getting into the high numbers—94—95—96 ("better count sheep than do this"). You are becoming a little tired, for it is awfully monotonous, and are getting to be a little mixed up and don't know the next number, so while you are foggily trying to remember it, your movement becomes slower and slower, until someone suddenly says, "Wake up, it's eight o'clock, breakfast is almost over."

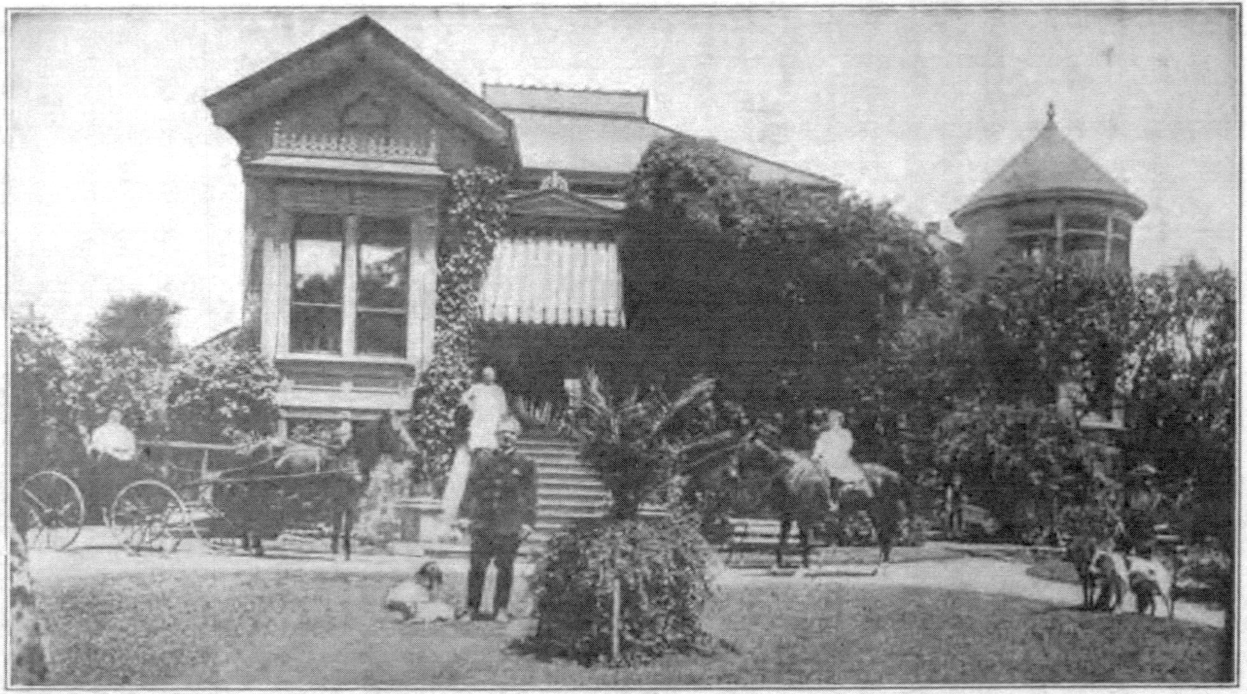

"Buena Vista," Home of Sanford Bennett, Alameda, California

In Conclusion

I HAVE now described, as fully and clearly as I am capable of doing, the methods by which I have accomplished my physical rejuvenation, and why such a condition as mine, at seventy-two, is possible by the system I practice. There is no question of my success, and I know the same satisfactory results are possible for any one who will follow my example; but will you do so? The majority will say, "That man has some good ideas," and add, "I feel that I do need a methodical system of exercise, and when I have time I may take this up." You might as well say you have no time to eat or sleep. You can't be healthy unless you exercise. Health should be your first consideration. Financial success and other things are of secondary importance; for with health, strength and elasticity of body the chances of financial success are greatly increased. Without these attributes, the greatest financial success is of but little value.

How many of our brain workers—our business men and professional men—have sacrificed health and happiness by following the paradox, "I am too busy—I haven't time to take care of my health"? There is only one result to a life upon these lines—an early breakdown is inevitably certain. It is true that many have accomplished great wealth in exchange for their health, but have spent that wealth in vainly endeavoring to regain their former, but now wasted, physical vigor.

I don't decry financial success. Wealth is a very good thing to have; but the greatest financial success will not compensate for ill health. Better stop now, before it is too late, and take the time to make yourself strong, for otherwise you may be forced to attend your own funeral, brought about prematurely by lack of muscular activity and other violations of the laws of Nature.

Another objection often raised is, "I am too old." To this I have already made my answer. If I, a chronic dyspeptic at fifty, with adverse hereditary and physical conditions and unfavorable environments, have been able, by the simple methods I have described, to build myself up and to acquire the strength, elasticity of body, and vital energy I now possess, but never had in the best days of my youth, then you, too, can surely have the same success. You are not too old. Try it. Commence now, and you will succeed.

"Too much trouble"—that is the objection of a lazy person. If, by the same exertions for one year, you could be assured that you would receive $50,000, you would not think that too much trouble, but would esteem it the opportunity of your life. Yet the health and improved physical condition which would surely result from one year's systematic and persistent practice of the methods I have described, could not be purchased for that or any other sum.

It is true that to be in the best physical condition does require unremitting attention; but the end is worth the means, for the reward is health, strength, elasticity of body, and longevity—the real, the greatest, riches in the world. Just as engineers and expert machinists, employed to care for the intricate machinery of a great ocean steamship, are forever polishing up and looking after the various details of that machinery, that they may have its highest efficiency; so the complicated machinery of the human body must be assiduously and intelligently cared for, or it will surely deteriorate.

There is no "royal road to health." It cannot be bought; if you would possess it you must work for it. But the way is easy, the work not hard. As you lie comfortably in bed to-morrow morning, commence the practice of any one of the muscular contractions and relaxations I have described, and when you have learned that, take up the next. Finally you will have acquired the whole system, which you will find to be an easy, certain and inexpensive method of acquiring health. You will find all of the exercises easily learned. "DO IT NOW." Commence to-morrow morning.

Yours sincerely,

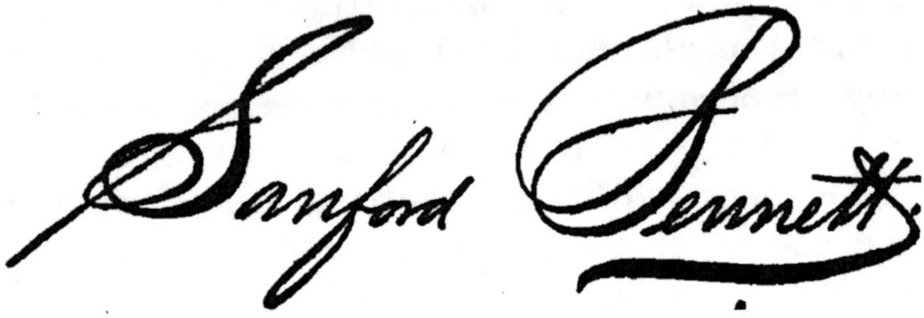

writings of Bernarr Macfadden (editor Physical Culture Magazine), which, with essays of other recognized authorities upon the science of health, strength, elasticity of body, good digestion and Nature's methods of obtaining a long life, without the use of drugs, constitute the five volumes of "Macfadden's Encyclopedia of Physical Culture." For in this valuable collection of information will be found the answers to the questions which have been propounded to me, as well as a vast amount of reliable data in the greatest of all sciences. The matter is alphabetically arranged for quick reference. It has all been carefully considered by Editor Macfadden, and is invaluable. There has never been anything like it published. That I may contribute my little help toward the advancement of the science of health and a long life without drugs, I have made an arrangement with the Physical Culture Publishing Company that any purchaser of a copy of OLD AGE—ITS CAUSE AND PREVENTION at the regular retail price of $1.50, shall be given a voucher for that amount, which will be accepted by them at its face value on account of the purchase of Macfadden's Encyclopedia of Physical Culture. In this way the information requested, but which I have failed to furnish, will be obtained quicker and probably in most cases will be more clearly presented than I could have done, even if I could have answered the questions, which I must admit have often been "beyond my pen." My advice is to read carefully my own experiences in getting young again at 72, which you will find in OLD AGE—ITS CAUSE AND PREVENTION, then buy Macfadden's Encyclopedia, read up your own case, be your own doctor, don't use any more drugs, and send me your thanks for "giving you the tip." Use the big books as a warehouse of reliable, valuable information, which you will surely need when you commence the study of the science of taking care of your body, by rational methods and without drugs, druggists, or drug store doctors. The investment I advise is the best you can make. I might not have time to give you the information required, and possibly I couldn't do it if I wanted to, but you are pretty sure to find it in that warehouse of information. You have my kindest wishes for your success in the art of getting young again and I would like to hear you have succeeded. Anyhow, I am positive you will be greatly benefited if you will take my advice in the matter.

Sincerely yours,

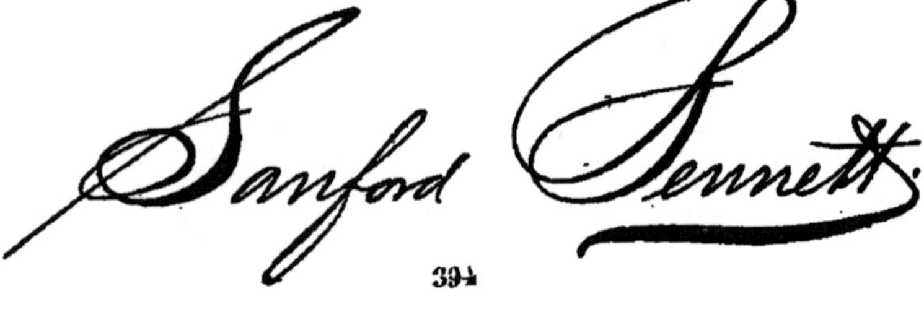

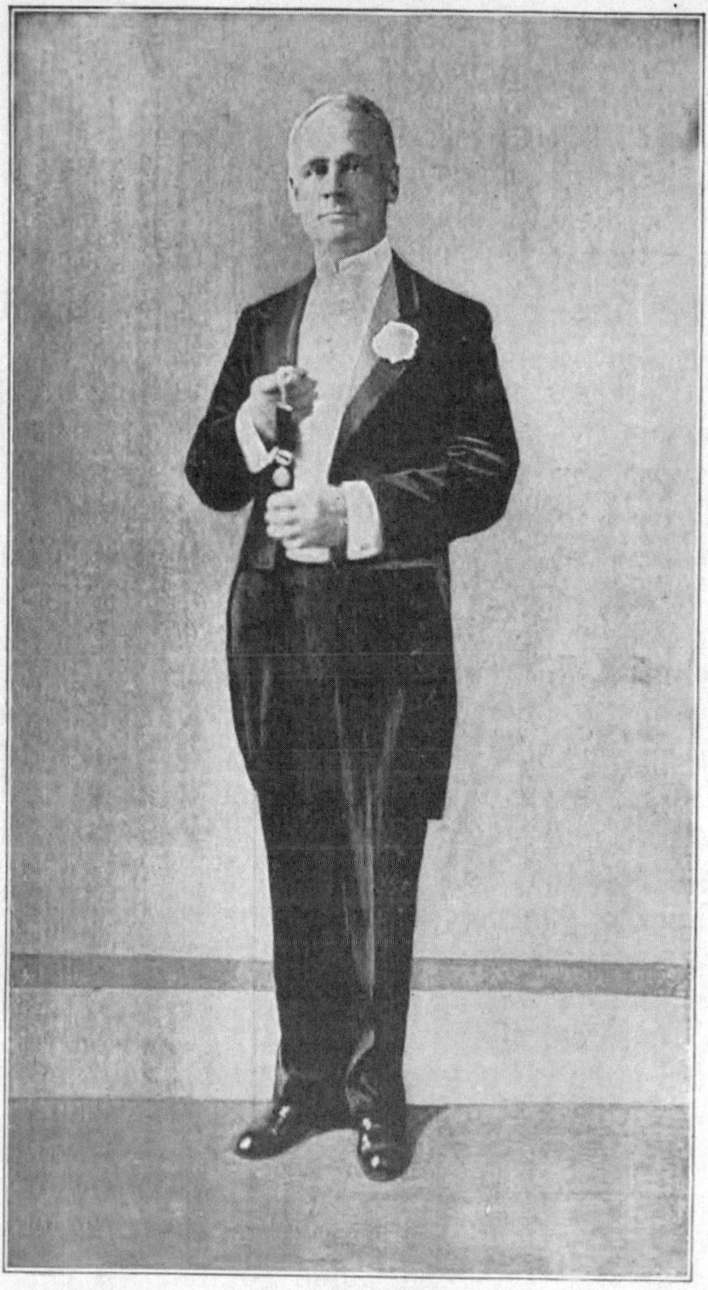

"I Move We Adjourn."

As to Questions That May Arise

IN my first book, entitled "Exercising in Bed," I told the story of my physical rejuvenation at 72, and described the simple means by which I have regained my physical youth at "over three score years and ten." Then I very rashly told the readers of that book that, if they did not clearly understand the methods I described, and would write to me, I would gladly explain any problems which I had solved in the science of getting young again. The result of that invitation has been such an avalanche of questions that I have been unable to answer a great many letters and must apologize to the writers for my apparent lack of good faith. In this new literary venture I had intended to answer all of those questions, but I find that space will not permit. As OLD AGE—ITS CAUSE AND PREVENTION is already a larger book than I had intended, I know that I should make good my promise, but I have not the time, even if I had the space. In this dilemma I have decided to do the next best thing; really the very best thing, and that is to refer the questioners to the remarkable compilation of the